Transvaginal Colour Doppler

Springer
*Berlin
Heidelberg
New York
Barcelona
Budapest
Hong Kong
London
Milan
Paris
Tokyo*

T.H. Bourne   E. Jauniaux
D. Jurkovic   (Eds.)

Transvaginal Colour Doppler

The Scientific Basis
and Practical Application
of Colour Doppler in Gynaecology

With Contributions by
S. Athanasiou, B. Bauer, R. Bicknell, J.E. Boultbee, T.H. Bourne,
G.J. Burton, S. Campbell, L.D. Cardozo, F.A. Chervenak, J.A. Cullinan,
F. Flam, A.C. Fleischer, H. Fox, R.W. Gill, K. Gruböck, E. Hacket,
J. Hustin, E. Jauniaux, D. Jurkovic, D. Kepple, V. Khullar, T. Loupas,
G. Moscoso, E.S. Newlands, K. Reynolds, G. Sharland,
I.P. van Splunder, C.V. Steer, A. Tailor, M. Toth, L. Valentin,
J.W. Wladimiroff

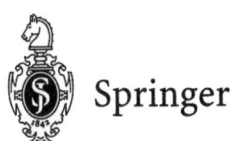 Springer

Tom Bourne MB. BS, Ph.D., MRCOG
Academic Department of Obstetrics & Gynaecology
King's College School of Medicine & Dentistry
Denmark Hill, London SE5 8RX
United Kingdom

Eric Jauniaux, M.D., Ph.D.
Academic Department of Obstetrics & Gynaecology
University College London Medical School
86–96 Chenies Mews, London WCIE 6HX
United Kingdom

Davor Jurkovic, M.D., Ph.D., MRCOG
Academic Department of Obstetrics & Gynaecology
King's College School of Medicine and Dentistry
Denmark Hill, London SE5 8RX
United Kingdom

With 97 Figures, Some in Colour

ISBN-13:978-3-642-79266-3   e-ISBN-13:978-3-642-79264-9
DOI: 10.1007/978-3-642-79264-9

Library of Congress Cataloging-in-Publication Data. Transvaginal colour Doppler:the scientific basis and practical applications of colour Doppler in gynaecology/Tom H. Bourne, Eric Jauniaux, Davor Jurkovic, eds.:with contributions by S. Athanasiou ... [et al.]. p. cm. Includes bibliographical references and index. ISBN-13:978-3-642-79266-3 (alk. paper)1.Transvaginal ultrasonography. 2. Doppler ultrasonography. I. Bourne, Tom H., 1959- . II. Jauniaux, E. III. Jurkovic, Davor, 1958- . IV. Athanasiou, S. [DNLM: 1. Genital Diseases, Female—ultrasonography. 2. Urogenital System—ultrasonography. 3. Prenatal Diagnosis. WP 141 T7713 1995] RG107.5.T73T72 1995 618.1'07543—dc20 DNLM/DLC for Library of Congress 95-2189

The use of general descriptive names, registered names, trademarks, etc. in this publication does not imply, even in the absence of a specific statement, that such names are exempt from the relevant protective laws and regulations and therefore free for general use.

Product liability: The publisher cannot guarantee the accuracy of any information about dosage and application contained in this book. In every individual case the user must check such information by consulting the relevant literature.

Typesetting: Best-set Typesetter Ltd., Hong Kong

SPIN: 10125527   23/3130/SPS – 5 4 3 2 1 0 – Printed on acid-free paper

Preface

Since the pioneering work of Donald and his first *Lancet* paper in 1958, the use of ultrasound in obstetrics and gynaecology has evolved rapidly. The introduction of grey scale techniques enhanced our ability to identify different tissues on the basis of their texture. However, it was the introduction of the linear array real-time scanner in the mid seventies that changed ultrasound from being an "eccentric art form" to a readily available and usable technique. This led to the first reports of the diagnosis of neural tube defects using ultrasound by Campbell, as well as the establishment of fetal biometry. In the midst of this activity the parallel development of the transvaginal probe by Kratochwill went almost unnoticed by most gynaecologists. Yet the application of this technique has since had a major impact on many areas of gynaecological practice, and on infertility in particular. Since the demonstration of transvaginal follicle aspiration, the vaginal route has become standard for most invasive ultrasound guided gynaecological procedures. The relatively new technical advance of transvaginal colour Doppler may potentially have just as great an impact. The introduction and use of transvaginal colour flow imaging has facilitated the study of vascular changes within the pelvis. The follicle and corpus luteum of the ovary and the endometrium of the uterus are the only areas in a normal adult body where angiogenesis (the development of new blood vessels) occurs to any significant extent; the same process occurs during the growth of carcinomas. The ability to recognise these early vascular changes with colour Doppler is facilitating the diagnosis of pelvic cancers as well as normal and abnormal ovarian and uterine function. It seems likely that this new technique will lead to a greater understanding of how vessel growth is involved in reproductive pathophysiology. The ability to monitor changes in vascularity may enable the development of methods to inhibit or enhance angiogenic activity in vivo.

There are problems to be overcome, however, before we should become overenthusiastic about this new technology. A brief review of the literature on the subject reveals a significant variation in results obtained by different authors. When we first published a series of ovarian tumours assessed with transvaginal colour Doppler, of 30 tumors studied there was one false negative and one false positive test result for the presence of ovarian carcinoma. The test was never likely to be perfect. At that time we thought low impedance flow was pathognomonic for the presence of carcinoma. Subsequently we observed that such flow patterns were a ubiquitous finding throughout many ovarian cycles, and not unusual even in postmenopausal ovaries. It has become clear that the classification of ovarian tumours in young women using transvaginal colour Doppler is difficult. Anyone who actually performs such scans themselves will be familiar with the wide variety of blood flow patterns that may be generated from premenopausal ovaries.

The wide variability in results encountered by many users of colour Doppler has led to confusion. In fact colour Doppler is neither as good as some workers proclaim nor as bad as others would have us believe. The truth lies somewhere in the middle. Used uncritically, in isolation and in inexperienced hands, transvaginal colour Doppler will be at best useless and at worst dangerous. One is reminded of a famous English photographer who observed that whilst there must be millions of SLR camaras in England, it was a shame that less than ten of the owners knew how to use them. Unfortunately, whilst obviously an exaggeration, the situation with colour Doppler machines is not so very different. The number of doctors who wish to learn colour Doppler having had little or no experience of B mode ultrasonography illustrates the problem.

Notwithstanding the limitations discussed in this book, when applied by expert operators and in a disciplined fashion, colour Doppler will add significantly to the diagnostic information available. We believe that there has been a tendency towards overenthusiasm and uncritical acceptance of transvaginal colour Doppler into clinical practice. This is unhelpful both for clinicians and patients, as well as for the technique itself. In this book we believe we have presented a realistic picture of the work that has been performed to date using this technique, whilst indicating possible applications in the future. We hope the reader will be left with a clear picture of what to believe and not believe when interpreting data related to colour Doppler, and a better understanding of what to expect from their equipment.

London, February 1995   TOM BOURNE
                                         ERIC JAUNIAUX
                                         DAVOR JURKOVIC

Contents

List of Contributors

ATHANASIOU, S., M.D., MRCOG
Academic Department of Obstetrics and Gynaecology,
King's College School of Medicine and Dentistry, Denmark Hill,
London SE5 8RX, United Kingdom

BAUER, B., M.D.
The Ovarian Screening and Gynaecological Scanning Unit,
Academic Department of Obstetrics and Gynaecology,
King's College School of Medicine and Dentistry, Denmark Hill,
London SE5 8RX, United Kingdom

BICKNELL, R., Ph.D.
Molecular Angiogenesis Group, Imperial Cancer Research Fund
Laboratories, Institute of Molecular Medicine,
University of Oxford, John Radcliffe Hospital, Headington,
Oxford OX3 9DU, United Kingdom

BOULTBEE, J.E., MRCP
Department of Radiology, Charing Cross Hospital,
Fulham Palace Road, London W6 8RF, United Kingdom

BOURNE, T.H., MB. BS, Ph.D, MRCOG
Ovarian Screening and Gynaecological Ultrasound Unit,
Academic Department of Obstetrics and Gynaecology,
King's College School of Medicine and Dentistry, Denmark Hill,
London SE5 8RX, United Kingdom

BURTON, G.J., M.D.
Department of Anatomy, University of Cambridge,
Downing Street, Cambridge CR2 3DY, United Kingdom

CAMPBELL, S., FRCOG
Academic Department of Obstetrics and Gynaecology,
King's College School of Medicine and Dentistry, Denmark Hill,
London SE5 8RX, United Kingdom

CARDOZO, L.D., M.D., FRCOG
Academic Department of Obstetrics and Gynaecology,
The Urogynaecology Unit, King's College Hospital,
Denmark Hill, London SE5 8RX, United Kingdom

CHERVENAK, F.A., M.D.
Department of Obstetrics and Gynaecology,
The New York Hospital, Cornell Medical Center,
525 East 68th Street, New York, NY 10021, USA

CULLINAN, J.A., M.D.
Department of Radiology and Radiological Sciences, Section
of Diagnostic Sonography, Vanderbilt University Medical Centre,
Nashville, TN 37232-2675, USA

FLAM, F., M.D.
Department of Obstetrics and Gynaecology, Karolinska Hospital,
17176 Stockholm, Sweden

FLEISCHER, A.C., M.D.
Department of Radiology and Radiological Sciences, Section
of Diagnostic Sonography, Vanderbilt University Medical Centre,
Nashville, TN 37232-2675, USA

FOX, H., M.D., FRCOG, FRC Path.
Department of Pathological Sciences, Stopford Building,
University of Manchester, Manchester M13 9PT, United Kingdom

GILL, R.W., Ph.D.
Ultrasonics Laboratory, Division of Radiophysics – CSIRO,
126 Greville Street, Chatswood NSW 2067, Australia

GRUBÖCK, K., M.D.
The Ovarian Screening and Gynaecological Scanning Unit,
Academic Department of Obstetrics and Gynaecology,
King's College School of Medicine and Dentistry, Denmark Hill,
London SE5 8RX, United Kingdom

HACKET, E., M.D.
The Ovarian Screening and Gynaecological Scanning Unit,
Academic Department of Obstetrics and Gynaecology,
King's College School of Medicine and Dentistry, Denmark Hill,
London SE5 8RX, United Kingdom

HUSTIN, J., M.D., Ph.D.
Institut de Morhologie Pathologique, Allée des Templiers,
41, 6280 Loverval, Belgium

JAUNIAUX, E., M.D., Ph.D.
   Academic Department of Obstetrics and Gynaecology, University
   College Hospital, Gower Street, London WI, United Kingdom

JURKOVIC, D., M.D., Ph.D., MRCOG
   Department of Obstetrics and Gynaecology, King's College School
   of Medicine and Dentistry, Denmark Hill, London SE5 8RX,
   United Kingdom

KEPPLE, D.M., RDMS
   Department of Radiology and Radiological Sciences, Section
   of Diagnostic Sonography, Vanderbilt University Medical Centre,
   Nashville, TN 37232-2675, USA

KHULLAR, V., MB. BS, BSc
   Academic Department of Obstetrics and Gynaecology,
   The Urogynaecology Unit, King's College Hospital,
   Denmark Hill, London SE5 9RS, United Kingdom

LOUPAS, T., DScENG
   Ultrasonics Laboratory, Division of Radiophysics – CSIRO,
   126 Greville Street, Chatswood NSW 2067, Australia

MOSCOSO, G., M.D., Ph.D.
   Early Human Development Research Unit, King's College School
   of Medicine and Dentistry, Denmark Hill, London SE5 8RX,
   United Kingdom

NEWLANDS, E.S., Ph.D., FRCP
   Department of Medical Oncology, Charing Cross Hospital,
   Fulham Palace Road, London W6 8RF, United Kingdom

REYNOLDS, K., FRCS (Ed), MRCOG
   Academic Department of Obstetrics and Gynaecology, King's
   College Hospital, Denmark Hill, London SE5 8RX,
   United Kingdom

SHARLAND, G., M.D., MRCP
   Department of Fetal Cardiology, Guy's Hospital, St. Thomas Street,
   London SE1 9RT, United Kingdom

VAN SPLUNDER, I.P., M.D.
   Department of Obstetrics and Gynaecology,
   Academic Hospital Rotterdam-Dijkzigt, Erasmus University
   Rotterdam, Dr. Molewaterplein 40, 3015 GD Rotterdam,
   The Netherlands

STEER, C.V., M.D., MRCOG
Department of Obstetrics and Gynaecology, Orpington Hospital,
Sevenoaks Road, Orpington, Kent BR6 9JU, United Kingdom

TAILOR, A., MB. BS
The Ovarian Screening Unit, Academic Department of Obstetrics
and Gynaecology, King's College Hospital, Denmark Hill, London
SE5 8RX, United Kingdom

TOTH, M., M.D.
Department of Obstetrics and Gynaecology, The New York
Hospital, Cornell Medical Center, 525 East 68th Street, New York,
NY 10021, USA

VALENTIN, L., M.D., Ph.D.
Department of Obstetrics and Gynaecology,
Malmö General Hospital, 21401 Malmö, Sweden

WLADIMIROFF, J.W., M.D., Ph.D.
Department of Obstetrics and Gynaecology,
Academic Hospital Rotterdam-Dijkzigt,
Erasmus University Rotterdam, Dr. Molewaterplein 40,
3015 GD Rotterdam, The Netherlands

I. General Principles

1. General Principles

Principles of Colour Doppler

T. Loupas and R.W. Gill

Introduction

Colour Doppler was originally developed in the mid-1980s, primarily as a technique for cardiac investigation [12]. Since then its uses have expanded considerably and cover almost every aspect of the circulation. This expansion is directly related to the fact that colour Doppler represents the most comprehensive form of ultrasonic imaging currently available, in the sense that it combines the anatomical information of high-resolution grey-scale B-mode scanning with a colour-coded map which depicts particular features of flow within a two-dimensional region of interest (the "colour box"). While B-mode ultrasound is an integral part of colour Doppler systems, a full description of its principles is clearly outside the scope of this chapter. In-depth treatment of this subject can be found in a number of standard books, such as those by Kremdau [7], McDicken [9] and Hykes et al. [6]. We will focus instead on the flow aspects of colour Doppler by examining the underlying physical principles which enable motion to be recorded by means of pulsed ultrasound, the technical aspects of producing flow images in real time, the controls of typical instruments and how they affect performance as well as a number of artefacts which require consideration in order to avoid misinterpretation.

Fundamental Concepts

Colour Doppler is an elaborate form of pulsed-wave (PW) Doppler and, therefore, relies on the same principle as spectral PW Doppler to detect motion, namely the gradual translation of the echoes received from moving targets between successive pulse transmissions (Fig. 1). By recording the value of the echoes received from a given depth each time a pulse is transmitted, a sequence of samples known as the Doppler signal is obtained. Motion in the vicinity of the fixed depth range gate will be manifested in the form of a time-varying Doppler signal, whose frequency f_D is given by the familiar Doppler equation

$$f_D = \frac{2 f_{RF} v \cos\theta}{c}$$

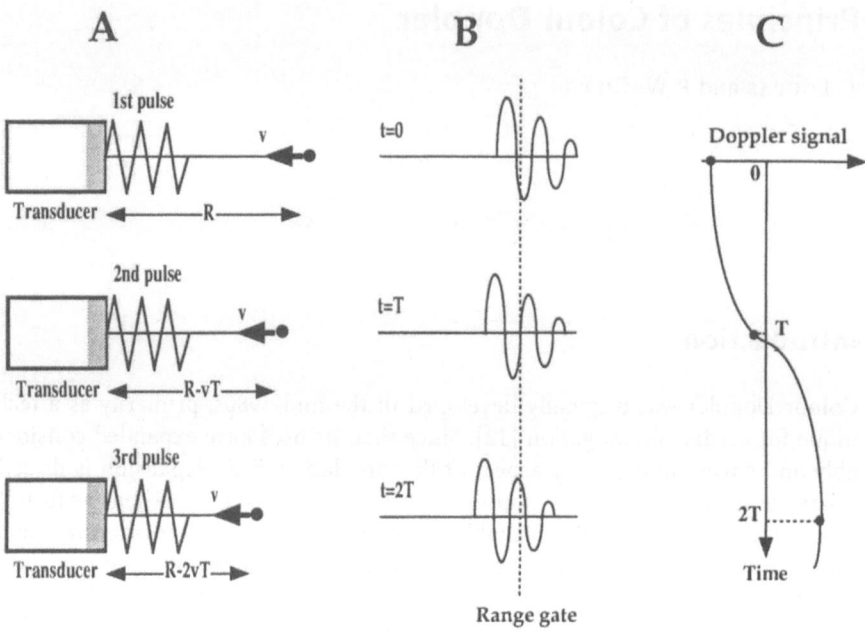

Fig. 1A–C. Simplified illustration of a target moving towards the transducer with velocity v and interrogated by an ultrasound pulse every T seconds, i.e. pulse repetition frequency (PRF) is $1/T$ Hz. Between two pulse transmissions the target moves closer to the transducer by a distance vT (**A**). This gradual translation is also evident on the reflected RF echoes received by the transducer (**B**). Range gating (the process of waiting for an appropriate time interval to receive echoes from a specific depth) detects a time-varying signal, known as the Doppler signal, whose frequency is proportional to the velocity of motion v relative to the transducer

where f_{RF} is the frequency of the incident pulse, c is the speed of sound in the medium, v is the velocity of the moving target and θ represents the Doppler angle, i.e. the angle between the direction of motion and the ultrasound beam.

The Doppler angle is of critical importance, since the quantity actually measured is the component of the velocity along the beam, as Fig. 2 illustrates. The same figure emphasises the well-known principle that positive and negative Doppler frequencies correspond to motion towards and away from the transducer, respectively. The Doppler equation implies that motion at right angles to the beam (θ, 90°) results in a zero Doppler frequency (cos 90°, 0). However, a non-constant Doppler signal of measurable power can still be detected in this situation [4]. It simply contains equal positive and negative frequencies which cancel each other out, resulting in the *mean* Doppler frequency being equal to zero. In such regions, spectral PW Doppler will record traces which are symmetrical with respect to the baseline on the spectral display, while a colour Doppler instrument measuring the mean Doppler frequency will colour the region black. The angle dependence of Doppler systems should always be kept in mind to avoid ambiguities and misinterpretation in cases such as those highlighted in Fig. 3.

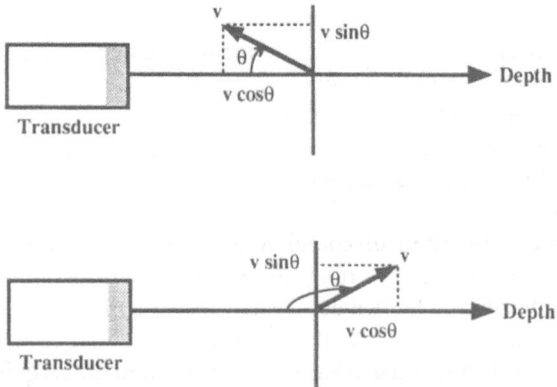

Fig. 2. A velocity v along an arbitrary direction can be decomposed into an axial part along the beam ($v \cos \theta$), which is the component measured by Doppler, and a lateral part at right angles to the beam ($v \sin \theta$). The sign of the Doppler frequency is determined by $\cos \theta$. Hence, it is positive for motion towards the transducer ($\cos \theta$ goes from 1 to 0 as θ varies from 0° to 90°) and negative for motion away from the transducer ($\cos \theta$ goes from 0 to −1 as θ varies from 90° to 180°)

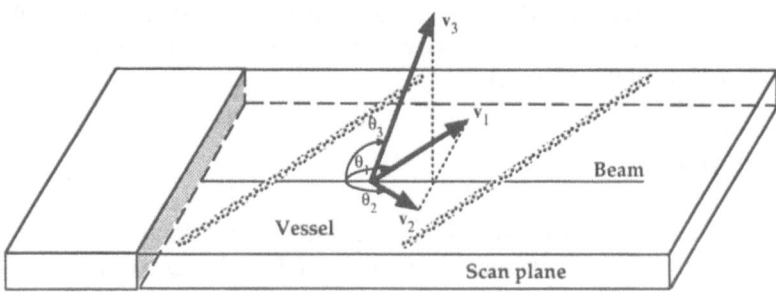

Fig. 3. Three velocities (v_1 parallel to the vessel walls, v_2 at an angle to the walls, and v_3 lying outside the scan plane) which have the same component along the ultrasound beam and, therefore, result in the same Doppler frequency

   The three-dimensional region from which Doppler signals are detected, for a given position of the range gate, is called the sample volume of Doppler systems. The axial extent of the sample volume is directly related to the length of the transmitted pulse, while the other two dimensions are determined by the lateral beam width and the thickness of the scanning plane. None of these quantities is under direct user control in colour Doppler, although it should be remembered that instruments tend to transmit longer pulses as the depth of penetration increases to compensate for the effect of increased attenuation [3].

   Since the vessel region encompassed by the sample volume generally contains targets (red blood cells) moving with different velocities, and possibly in different directions, real Doppler signals consist of a range of frequencies, rather than the pure sinusoid depicted in Fig. 1c. The value and relative power of each frequency component (i.e. the Doppler spectrum) can be estimated by means of mathematical techniques such as the Fourier transform [5]. This is the most complete representation of the information contained in the Doppler signal. In the case of colour Doppler, however, where it is not feasible to perform full spectral analysis for each point of the colour box (both from a computational and an ergonomic point of view), specific features describing particular aspects of the Doppler spectrum are measured and displayed instead.

Although the pulsed-mode operation of colour and spectral PW Doppler systems offers the highly desirable property of range discrimination, it also introduces a potentially important limitation known as aliasing. This is a direct consequence of the fact that a dynamic event, such as the motion of red blood cells, is observed only each time a pulse is transmitted. Aliasing occurs beyond the Nyquist limit, when the absolute value of the Doppler frequency exceeds half the rate of observation (i.e. the pulse repetition frequency, PRF). By making use of the Doppler equation, an equivalent condition for velocities can be formulated:

$$\text{Aliasing} \rightarrow |f_D| > \frac{PRF}{2} \rightarrow |v| > \frac{PRFc}{4f_{RF}\cos\theta}$$

Aliasing causes Doppler frequencies outside the range −PRF/2 to PRF/2 to wrap around so that, for example, a Doppler frequency slightly higher than PRF/2 will be recorded as a value just above −PRF/2 (see [2, 13] for more details on aliasing and the other concepts in this section).

Technical Aspects

Colour Doppler is an inherently two-dimensional technique. The challenge here is to extend the single sample volume of spectral PW Doppler to typically tens of thousands of sample volumes, so that particular aspects of flow can be measured and displayed in real time over the entire region of interest. Acquiring and processing multiple sample volumes along a fixed line of sight is relatively straightforward by means of multigating, i.e. by sampling the information received from a given line of sight at a number of incremental times corresponding to many adjacent range gates. After several pulses (minimum three and typically eight to 16) have been transmitted, an adjacent line of sight is interrogated by the same number of pulses, and this process is repeated until the entire region of interest has been scanned. The B-mode information required to form the grey-scale image can be acquired either after each colour line acquisition has been completed or by a separate sweep at the end of the colour frame capture. Note that different pulse lengths are generally used during the B-mode and colour Doppler transmissions (Doppler systems require considerably longer pulses to compensate for the poor signal-to-noise ratio due to the weak scattering nature of blood) and that most of the acquisition time per frame is devoted to colour Doppler, since B-mode requires only one pulse per line. As can be deduced from Table 1, high colour frame rates

Table 1. Step-by-step derivation of the colour frame rate

Time required for one transmit/receive cycle	$\dfrac{2R}{c}$
Time required for one colour acquisition per line of sight	$\dfrac{2RN}{c}$
Time required for one colour frame	$\dfrac{2RNLW}{c}$
Colour frame rate	$\dfrac{c}{2RNLW}$

c is the speed of sound, R the maximum depth of penetration, N the number of transmitted pulses per colour line, while L and W denote the line density and width of the colour box, respectively (i.e. the product LW gives the number of lines per colour box).

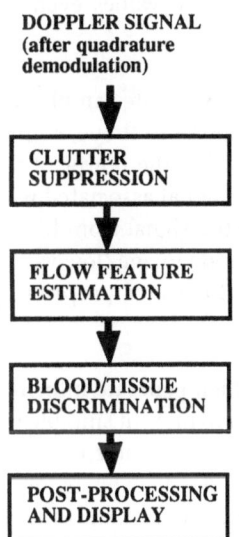

DOPPLER SIGNAL
(after quadrature demodulation)

CLUTTER SUPPRESSION

FLOW FEATURE ESTIMATION

BLOOD/TISSUE DISCRIMINATION

POST-PROCESSING AND DISPLAY

Fig. 4. Stages through which the Doppler signal passes. This chain is preceded by quadrature demodulation, a processing operation which takes the Doppler signal to a form suitable for extracting not only the magnitude of the Doppler frequency but also its sign, which reveals whether flow is towards or away from the transducer

can be achieved by reducing one or more of the following parameters: depth of penetration, number of pulses, line density and width of the colour box.

Figure 4 illustrates a typical colour Doppler processing chain. Each stage of this chain is briefly described below:

Clutter Suppression. Since the sample volume occupies a three-dimensional region, instead of the ideal case of being infinitely small, the received signal generally contains a significant contribution from the surrounding tissue (clutter), whose power is typically 100–100 000 times higher than that of the blood component. However, the fact that clutter is due to stationary or slowly moving tissue means that the corresponding Doppler signal tends to have a predominantly low-frequency content, which can be removed, at least partially, by means of filters which allow only the high Doppler frequencies associated with blood flow to pass through.

Flow Feature Estimation. The most common feature extracted from the clutter-suppressed Doppler signal is its mean frequency, which corresponds to the average axial velocity within the sample volume. Another feature is the variance of the Doppler spectrum, which provides an indication of the range of velocities inside the sample volume and can therefore be used as an indicator of turbulence. Although both features capture particular aspects of the Doppler spectrum, they are estimated in a computationally efficient manner directly from the Doppler signal, without the need to perform spectral analysis. A third feature, which has recently gained considerable prominence, is the power of the Doppler signal. For blood regions, this quantity is related to the number of moving red blood cells within the sample volume and has the advantage of producing non-zero values even for Doppler angles near 90°, as explained in the previous section.

Blood/Tissue Discrimination. The function of this stage is to separate sample volumes which contain mostly blood from those which correspond to tissue, so that only flow regions are colour coded. The main criterion used is the power of the Doppler signal since, after clutter suppression, the Doppler signal associated with tissue contains only noise, which tends to be weaker than the signal from blood. However, other criteria such as the echogenicity of the B-mode image (low values imply blood while high values signify tissue) and more sophisticated proprietary techniques are also used.

Post-processing and Display. Unlike the previous stages which generate information, this module manipulates already available information to make it suitable for display. It performs spatial and temporal smoothing to reduce the noisiness and improve the appearance of the Doppler data, interpolation and scan conversion, so that the low-resolution colour Doppler values can be superimposed onto the B-mode image grid, and colour coding of the selected flow features for those sample volumes classified as blood.

Instrument Controls

Although most instruments offer presets which adjust various operating parameters and controls to match the current clinical application, colour Doppler remains a highly interactive modality which relies heavily on the user's judgement and expertise to optimise the image. The most important controls are:

Colour Box. The area from which colour Doppler information is acquired is under the control of the user, who can adjust its position and dimensions so that it fully encompasses the vessels of interest. The width of the box has a significant effect on the instrument's performance, since the line density and/or frame rate must be reduced as the box becomes wider in order to satisfy the physical constraints highlighted by Table 1. The box height affects the instrument's axial resolution due to computational rather than physical constraints, in the sense that many instruments subdivide the colour box axially into a fixed number of sample volumes, irrespective of its height. Hence, the shorter the box, the better the axial resolution.

Steering Angle. This feature is applicable only to linear transducers. It allows the user to control the direction of the Doppler beam depending on the orientation of the vessels of interest and solves, at least partially, the conflicting beam direction requirements of B-mode and Doppler techniques (structures are imaged best at right angles of incidence, while Doppler requires that the beam and flow direction are as parallel as possible).

Flow Feature and Scale Selection. The options offered are to display the mean frequency, a combination of mean frequency and variance or the power of the Doppler signal. When the selected feature is the mean frequency, the scale can be expressed either in frequency (kHz) or velocity (cm/s) units, where the conversion between the two is performed using the Doppler equation and assuming an angle of 0°. Adjusting the scale affects the PRF used by the system. For example, if the maximum frequency on the scale is 2.5 kHz, the PRF is equal to 5 kHz (remember that for a given PRF, the non-aliased values occupy the range from minus to plus PRF/2). Obviously, setting the scale too low may result in severe aliasing. On the contrary, a very high scale will allocate almost the same colour shade to all velocities found in the vessel and may even result in loss of colour.

Clutter Suppression. This control is of critical importance. An aggressive setting (a very high frequency filter cut-off) may eliminate regions of slow flow, while a very low cut-off may allow the tissue clutter to obscure the Doppler signal from blood, so that the colour display is predominantly due to tissue motion instead of blood flow. More sophisticated clutter suppression techniques are capable of eliminating tissue motion while allowing slow flow to be visualised, but this is usually done at the expense of increased computations and, consequently, reduced frame rate.

Colour Gain. This control has a direct effect on the tissue/blood discrimination which, as was explained in the previous section, is performed mostly on the basis of the strength of the Doppler signal associated with each pixel. Therefore, increasing the gain may allow visualisation of true flow which had previously been below the system threshold. At the same time, excessive gain will also cause tissue pixels, whose Doppler signal is entirely due to noise, to exceed the threshold, resulting in a large number of colour dots randomly distributed throughout the image.

Acoustic Output. Unlike colour gain, which amplifies the received signal and the noise equally, the acoustic output control determines the power transmitted into the body. Consequently, it can increase the received signal preferentially over noise, resulting in a higher signal-to-noise ratio and improving the detectability of weak flow. However, it is imperative that the current safety guidelines [1] are always obeyed and that extra caution is exercised during foetal examinations.

Number of Pulses. Setting the system to transmit more pulses per colour line represents an effective way of improving both clutter suppression and the quality of the calculated flow features. Unfortunately, this increases the acquisition time proportionally and, consequently, lowers either the frame rate or the line density.

Smoothing. While a significant amount of averaging is performed by colour Doppler instruments, both within the same frame (spatial smoothing) and between successive frames (temporal smoothing, or persistence), the user can commonly adjust only the temporal aspect. Heavy frame averaging may improve the definition of flow regions but, at the same time, degrades temporal resolution and, therefore, is inappropriate in the context of transient flow events such as flow reversals and highly pulsatile flow.

Artefacts

A number of artefacts are associated with colour Doppler, which may cause misinterpretation of the underlying haemodynamics [8, 10, 14].

Aliasing, a characteristic of all pulsed Doppler systems, does not usually represent a serious limitation for colour Doppler, due to the qualitative nature of this modality. It may even be of help in flagging the presence of high velocities, provided it is not too severe (i.e. Doppler frequencies do not exceed ±3 PRF/2, so that they are wrapped only once around the primary range of −PRF/2 to PRF/2). It should also be straightforward to distinguish aliasing from flow reversal, since in the former case there is an abrupt colour transition from one end of the colour scale to the other (Fig. 5), while in the latter case there is a dark colour boundary (zero flow) between colour regions corresponding to opposite directions. Aliasing can be corrected by increasing the PRF (either by reducing the maximum penetration depth or expanding the frequency/velocity scale), shifting the baseline (provided that aliasing is not too severe) so that the scale is reallocated to, say, 0 to PRF instead of the default range −PRF/2 to PRF/2, obtaining a Doppler angle closer to 90°, or using a lower frequency probe.

The angle dependence of Doppler systems must always be kept in mind to resolve potential ambiguities. Common manifestations of this dependence include flow which appears non-uniform, or even at different directions, when the vessel is curved or is scanned by a curved transducer (Fig. 5), complex colour patterns when the flow is not parallel to the vessel walls, and lack of flow visualisation at angles around 90°.

Another, more subtle, source of ambiguity is the fact that a colour frame, instead of being an instantaneous representation of flow throughout the region of

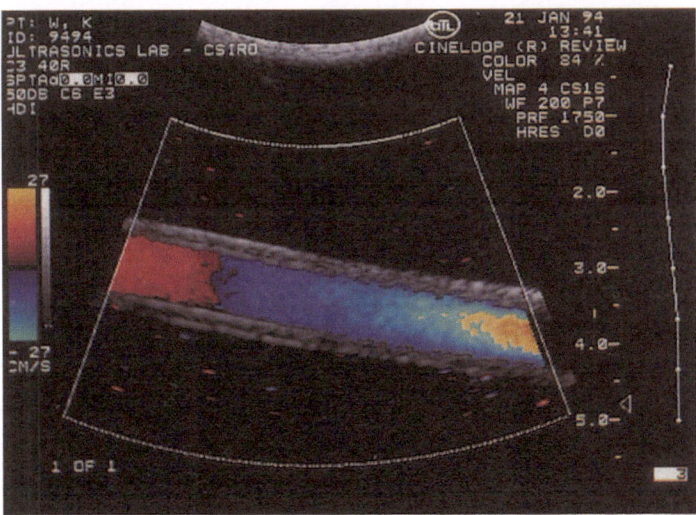

Fig. 5. Scan of constant flow through a tube, demonstrating the angle dependence of colour Doppler. Due to the curved scan format, the beam-to-vessel angle varies from less than 90° (flow towards the transducer, depicted as *red*) to a value well beyond 90° (flow away from the transducer, depicted as increasingly brighter shades of *blue* and leading eventually to aliasing). Also, note the poor colour definition when the beam is at right angles to the vessel and the presence of random colour dots in the background, due to noise

interest, is formed gradually on a line-by-line basis. Therefore, each part of the frame is captured at a different point of the cardiac cycle so that, for example, a flow reversal occurring throughout the vessel but during a very short time may be displayed as a localised event occupying only a particular area of the vessel lumen.

In general, it is important to remember that the presence or absence of flow in the colour image could well be of artefactual nature. Erroneously displayed flow may be due to tissue motion – "flash" artefact, multiple reflections (in which case a duplicate colour image of a vessel could appear deeper inside the body) or noise, especially in anechoic regions such as stationary fluid collections [11]. Also, colour may extend beyond the vessel boundaries due to a combination of wall motion, poor axial resolution and excessive colour gain. On the other hand, lack of flow may be due to a Doppler angle near 90°, excessive clutter suppression (which also tends to remove the signal from the slow-moving blood near the walls of large vessels), inappropriately high frequency/velocity scale or insufficient colour gain and power level. The presence or absence of flow should always be confirmed by means of spectral Doppler, since observing how the spectral trace varies with time is still the most reliable method of determining what represents true flow as well as identifying the vessel currently scanned.

References

1. Barnett SB, Kossoff G (eds) (1992) Special issue on WFUMB symposium on safety and standardisation in medical ultrasound. Ultrasound Med Biol 18: 731–810
2. Burns PN (1987) The physical principles of Doppler and spectral analysis. J Clin Ultrasound 15: 567–590
3. Deane CR, Forsberg F, Thomas N, Roberts VC (1991) Accuracy of colour Doppler ultrasound velocity measurements in small vessels. J Biomed Eng 13: 249–254
4. Dickerson KS, Newhouse VL, Tortoli P, Guidi G (1993) Comparison of conventional and transverse Doppler sonograms. J Ultrasound Med 12: 497–506
5. Hoeks APG, Hennerici M, Reneman RS (1991) Spectral composition of Doppler signals. Ultrasound Med Biol 17: 751–760
6. Hykes D, Hendrick W, Starchman D (1992) Ultrasound physics and instrumentation. Mosby, St Louis
7. Kremkau FW (1989) Diagnostic ultrasound: principles, instrumentation and exercises. Saunders, Philadelphia
8. Kurjak A, Shalan H, Kupesic S, Predanic M, Zalud I, Breyer B, Jukic S (1993) Transvaginal colour Doppler sonography in the assessment of pelvic tumor vascularity. Ultrasound Obstet Gynecol 3: 137–154
9. McDicken WN (1991) Diagnostic ultrasonics: principles and use of instruments. Churchill Livingstone, Edinburgh
10. Mitchell DG (1990) Colour Doppler imaging: principles, limitations and artifacts. Radiology 177: 1–10
11. Mitchell DG, Burns P, Needleman L (1990) Colour Doppler artifact in anechoic regions. J Ultrasound Med 9: 255–260
12. Omoto R (ed) (1984) Colour atlas of two-dimensional Doppler echocardiography. Shirdan-To-Chiryo, Tokyo
13. Taylor KJW, Burns PN, Wells PNT (1988) Clinical applications of Doppler ultrasound. Raven, New York
14. Taylor KJW, Holland S (1990) Doppler US, part I: basic principles, instrumentation and pitfalls. Radiology 174: 297–307

Angiogenesis

K. Reynolds and R. Bicknell

Introduction

Transvaginal colour Doppler imaging allows us to study the complex and dynamic vascular system that is the human female pelvis. Physiological or pathological angiogenesis may transform this vascular map, and this section will therefore outline our current understanding of angiogenesis as it occurs in the female pelvis. As physiological angiogenesis has been extensively studied in the ovary, the emphasis is on this organ. The vascular system in the foetus, the vascular anatomy of the pelvis and the pathophysiology of early placentation are discussed in later chapters and will not be dealt with here.

The Concept of Angiogenesis

Angiogenesis is the formation of new blood vessels; the term was first used in 1935 to describe this process in the placenta [1]. Thirty years later, Folkman initiated studies that showed that tumours do not grow beyond a size of 2–3 mm^3 unless they are able to attract the growth of new capillaries from the existing vascular network. In 1972, on the basis of these studies, he proposed the somewhat controversial hypothesis that solid tumours are angiogenesis dependent [2]. Now, 20 years later it is widely accepted that angiogenesis is an obligatory event for the sustained growth of solid tumours. This has been reviewed by Folkman [3]. It is also recognised that inhibition of this process might provide an opportunity for therapeutic intervention not just in the management of malignancies, but also of the many other non-neoplastic diseases characterised by persistent angiogenesis, such as diabetic retinopathy and rheumatoid arthritis.

Angiogenesis is an essential part of wound healing, growth and development, but in these cases it is highly regulated, as opposed to the persistent unregulated process that occurs in pathological states including cancer. In most healthy adult tissues, endothelial cells have a low mitotic rate and form a very quiescent population. The tissues of the female reproductive system are the only sites in the healthy adult human body where rapid proliferation of endothelial cells and angiogenesis occur. This is not surprising when one considers the cyclical growth and regression of the ovary and endometrium and the marked alterations in blood flow that accompany these changes [4]. These changes may be detected by transvaginal colour Doppler. Those practising this technique must therefore have an appreciation of the dynamic nature of the pelvic vascular system in health and disease if they are to interpret the images obtained and to differentiate physiological and pathological conditions.

The Angiogenic Process

The angiogenic process can been studied in detail by implanting small tumour pellets into the cornea of a rabbit which has been anaesthetized. This results in the formation of new blood vessels, which grow towards the tumour, the vessels regressing when the pellet is removed. Using this technique, the sequential steps in the angiogenic process have been identified [5]. New blood vessels arise from post-capillary venules in response to an angiogenic stimulus. Proteolysis of the basement membrane and degradation of the interstitial matrix at the site of new vessel formation is followed by the migration of endothelial cells towards the angiogenic stimulus. The cells align themselves to form a capillary bud, which is canalised to form a tubule. Proliferation of endothelial cells occurs proximal to the tip of this capillary bud, which joins with an adjacent bud to form a capillary loop and blood begins to flow.

The component steps in the process described above can be studied in vitro by growing endothelial cells in tumour-conditioned media. In these circumstances the cells will migrate, proliferate and form hollow tubes and branches, thus producing a capillary network in a petri dish [6]. These in vitro studies together with in vivo methods of inducing neovascularisation in the rabbit or rodent cornea and the chick embryo provide bioassays in which the activity of candidate angiogenic factors can be assessed.

When the search for angiogenic factors began it was presumed that such factors would have angiogenic activity in in vivo assays and would also be mitogenic and chemotactic for endothelial cells. Over the last 10 years, the list of angiogenic factors has rapidly expanded but few have been assessed in each assay, leaving an incomplete picture of the role of different factors in angiogenesis. Acidic (aFGF) and basic (bFGF) fibroblast growth factors are members of a family of sequence-related growth factors, all of which are potentially angiogenically active. Both are mitogenic and chemotactic for endothelial cells, and bFGF is the most potent stimulator of angiogenesis identified to date [7]. Other angiogenic peptides which are also endothelial cell mitogens include the epidermal growth factor (EGF) family, transforming growth factor (TGF) alpha [8] and vascular endothelial growth factor (VEGF) [9]. By comparison, angiogenin and platelet-derived endothelial cell growth factor (PD-ECGF) are not mitogens and, furthermore, TGF-β, tumour necrosis factor (TNF) alpha and interleukins-1 and -6 are actually endothelial cell growth inhibitors [10, 11]. This apparent paradox can be resolved if there are multiple pathways all of which result in angiogenesis. Angiogenic factors such as bFGF, which stimulate endothelial cells to migrate, divide and form new blood vessels, can stimulate neovascularisation directly.

However, inhibitory factors such as TGF-β can achieve the same end result by causing inflammation or by inducing the production of secondary factors which have a direct mitogenic effect. It has been shown that the neovascularisation produced by TGF-β in the rabbit cornea is accompanied by an inflammatory response [12]. The complexity of the angiogenic process is further complicated by the fact that there are numerous other non-polypeptide factors which have angiogenic activity.

Angiogenesis in the Female Reproductive System

The follicle and corpus luteum of the ovary and the endometrium of the uterus are the only sites in the healthy adult body where angiogenesis occurs to any significant extent. Thus, the ovary provides a model of physiological angiogenesis which can be compared with the pathological angiogenesis that occurs in ovarian cancer.

The pattern of neovascularisation around the developing follicle and corpus luteum can be visualised using an injection – corrosion technique which produces three-dimensional vascular casts of the ovary which are then observed with scanning electron microscopy [13, 14]. The characteristic vascular pattern starts as a simple capillary network around the primary follicles. With follicular development, a multilayered and complicated vascular system develops surrounding the follicles, the largest vascular network being that around the Graafian follicle. Just before rupture, marked dilatation of the vessels occurs and the new blood vessels become "leaky". Angiogenesis in the follicle is limited to the theca, but following follicular rupture the thecal vessels invade the granulosa layer to give rise to the luteal vascular network [13–16].

Follicles and corpora lutea have been shown to possess angiogenic activity in the rabbit cornea and chick chorioallantoic membrane assays, and the angiogenic activity of the former appears to be enhanced by gonadotrophin administration [17]. This effect is probably produced by the release of angiogenic factors from ovarian cells in response to gonadotrophic stimulation. Medium conditioned by granulosa cells is mitogenic and that conditioned by luteal cells is chemotactic for endothelial cells [17].

It has been shown that angiogenic activity is present in primate endometrium and that this activity is cyclical and associated with changes in systemic levels of ovarian steroids [18, 19]. Oestrogen and progesterone are presumed responsible for endometrial angiogenesis during the menstrual cycle. However, neither has intrinsic angiogenic activity. Indeed, the endothelial cells of the endometrium are oestrogen receptor negative [20], and it follows that the angiogenic response to oestrogen must come from the oestrogen receptor-positive epithelium or stromal component of the endometrium. While several angiogenic factors or their messenger ribonucleic acids (RNA) have been detected in endometrial tissue [21, 22], including VEGF, EGF, TGF-α [23] and bFGF [24], precisely which factors play a role in endometrial angiogenesis remains to be clarified.

Angiogenesis and Colour Doppler Imaging

Angiogenesis results in the formation of new capillary blood vessels. It would therefore be reasonable to assume that, if colour Doppler was sensitive enough to detect flow in these capillaries, it would also detect alterations in vascular patterns in the ovary at different time points in the menstrual cycle. This hypothesis was tested by using transvaginal ultrasound and colour Doppler imaging to assess intra-ovarian blood flow in relation to ovarian morphology and function during the periovulatory period (see the chapter by Bourne et al. on "Ovulation and the Periovulatory Follicle"). In the initial studies of 11 women (ten with apparently normal ovarian cycles), colour was first observed in the dominant follicle in the late follicular phase of the cycle. It was not detectable in the early follicular phase, even though angiogenesis is known to occur at this time. The velocity of blood flow in the vessels identified by colour Doppler imaging tended to increase approximately 29 h before the time of follicular rupture, and this rise continued for at least 72 h after the formation of the corpus haemorrhagicum.

Although we know that angiogenesis occurs in the early follicular phase of the cycle, it is possible that at this time the density of blood vessels is too low to allow detection of blood flow in neovascular areas. It is also conceivable that, with advances in technology and greater sensitivity of colour Doppler imaging, new blood flow will be identified at earlier time points in the cycle. The dramatic rise in peak systolic velocity observed is consistent with the marked dilatation of new blood vessels noted just before follicular rupture in studies of corrosion casts of ovarian follicles [13, 14] (see above). In particular, this rise in peak systolic velocity prefaced follicular rupture in the case in which rupture was actually observed as it occurred. The "fuzziness" of the pulsed Doppler waveform noted after follicular rupture might be explained by the "leakiness" of the vessels observed in corrosion casts in the periovulatory period [13, 14], although numerous other explanations are available. It would not be unreasonable to conclude that colour Doppler imaging can detect neovascular flow.

Studies on the use of colour Doppler imaging to differentiate between benign and malignant ovarian tumours in clinical practice and in screening programmes are encouraging (see the chapter by Bourne et al. on "The Study of Ovarian Tumours"). These studies show that malignant ovarian tumours are generally characterized by areas of high-velocity, low-resistance blood flow, whereas most benign tumours are not. Although it has been suggested that the pattern of colour is "patchier" in malignancy [25], the waveforms generated in these cases are not at the present time distinguishable from those found in the periovulatory ovary or corpus luteum, which might suggest that here too we are studying neovascular blood flow. However, many studies have shown that tumour implants are supplied not just by new blood vessels, but also by vessels recruited from the pre-existing host vasculature [26]. It is therefore possible that blood flow in these host vessels, which are probably consistently vasodilated, could produce the typical high-velocity, low-resistance waveforms seen in ovarian cancer.

It is not yet clear why certain benign tumours have the same features as malignant tumours when imaged by transvaginal colour Doppler. In ovarian endometriosis it is reasonable to assume that angiogenesis occurs as part of the accompanying inflammatory process, thus producing the typical waveforms associated with cancer. However, there are numerous other benign tumours that are not associated with inflammation that have these features. As angiogenesis is associated with progression from hyperplasia to neoplasia [27], it might be postulated that such tumours are at greater risk of malignant transformation. However, the existence of such a phenomenon in benign ovarian tumours has never been proven.

Future Prospects

Angiogenesis is an essential component of numerous physiological and pathological processes in the female pelvis. The potential for research in this area to produce novel approaches to the management of infertility, contraception and cancer is enormous.

The vascular density of breast tumours has been shown to correlate with prognosis [28]. As yet, studies on vascular density in ovarian tumours have not been done. If a correlation with malignancy or prognosis or both exists in ovarian cancer, there is a possibility that advances in technology will permit an accurate assessment of vascular density using transvaginal colour Doppler imaging. Such a non-invasive approach to diagnosis and assessment of prognosis would obviate the need for laparotomy, which is already pertinent in cases of benign disease but will become relevant to the management of ovarian cancer when alternatives to surgical treatment become available.

Recently, it was observed that there was a significant difference between the expression of mRNA for PD-ECGF between benign and malignant ovarian tumours [25]. It had already been shown that this angiogenic factor had thymidine phosphorylase activity [10], suggesting that enzyme inhibition might be of therapeutic benefit. Furthermore, it provides an opportunity for targeting chemotherapy in ovarian cancer as thymidine phosphorylase activates a pro-drug of 5-fluorouracil [29].

However, attempting to prevent tumour angiogenesis by targeting angiogenic factors is likely to be difficult: the already great and ever increasing number of angiogenic factors known, compounded by a lack of understanding of controlling mechanisms and interactions, indicates the difficulty of pursuing this approach at the present time. Furthermore, as tumours are supported by vasculature recruited from the host, inhibition of angiogenesis alone may not be adequate. Other approaches which exploit abnormal tumour vasculature are currently under investigation [29].

References

1. Hertig AT (1935) Angiogenesis in the early human chorion and in the primary placenta of the macaque monkey. Contrib Embryol 25: 39–81
2. Folkman J (1972) Anti-angiogenesis: new concept for therapy of solid tumors. Ann Surg 175: 409–416
3. Folkman J (1990) What is the evidence that tumors are angiogenesis dependent? J Natl Cancer Inst 82: 4–6
4. Ford S, Regnolds LP, Mugness RR (1982) Blood flow to the uterine and ovarian vascular beds of gilts during the estrous cycle and early pregnancy. Biol Reprod 27: 878–885
5. Ausprunk HA, Folkman J (1977) Migration and proliferation of endothelial cells in preformed and newly formed blood vessels during tumor angiogenesis. Microvasc Res 14: 53–65
6. Folkman J, Handenschild CC, Zetter BR (1979) Long-term culture of capillary endothelial cells. Proc Natl Acad Sci USA 76: 5217–5221
7. Klagsbrun M, D'Amore PA (1991) Regulators of angiogensis. Annu Rev Physiol 53: 217–239
8. Schrieber AB, Winkler ME, Derynck R (1986) Transforming growth factor-α: a more potent angiogenic mediator than epidermal growth factor. Science 232: 1250–1253
9. Tischer E, Gospodarowicz D, Mitchell R, et al (1989) Vascular endothelial growth factor: a new member of the platelet-derived growth factor gene family. Biochem Biophys Res Commun 165: 1198–1206
10. Moghaddam A, Bicknell R (1992) Expression of platelet-derived endothelial cell growth factor in Escherichia coli and confirmation of its thymidine phosphorylase activity. Biochemistry 31: 12141–12146
11. Bicknell R, Harris AL (1991) Novel growth regulatory factors and tumour angiogenesis. Eur J Cancer 27(6): 781–785
12. Folkman J, Klagsbrun M (1987) Angiogenic factors. Science 235: 442–447
13. Kanzaki H, Okamura H, Okuda Y (1982) Scanning electron microscopic study of rabbit ovarian follicle microvasculature using resin injection-corrosion casts. J Anat 134: 697–704
14. Murakami T, Ikebuchi Y, Ohtsuka A, et al (1988) The blood vascular wreath of rat ovarian follicle, with special reference to its changes in ovulation and luteinization: a scanning electron microscopic study of corrosion casts. Arch Histol Cytol 51: 299–313
15. Bassett DL (1943) the changes in the vascular pattern of the ovary of the albino rat during the estrous cycle. Am J Anat 73: 252–292
16. Brambell FWR (1956) Ovarian changes. In: Parkes AS (ed) Marshall's physiology of reproduction, vol 1 (1). Longmans and Green, London, pp 397–542
17. Koos R (1989) Potential relevance of angiogenic factors to ovarian physiology. Semin Reprod Endocrinol 7(1): 29–40
18. Markee JE (1940) Menstruation in intraocular endometrial transplants in the rhesus monkey. Contrib Embryol 77: 221–308
19. Abel MH (1985) Prostanoids and menstruation. In: Baird DT, Michie EA (eds) Mechanism of menstrual bleeding, vol 25. Raven, New York, pp 139–156 (Serono symposium 25)
20. Perrot-Applanat M, Groyer-Picard MT, Garcia E, et al (1988) Immunocytochemical demonstration of estrogen and progesterone receptors in muscle cells of uterine arteries in rabbits and humans. Endocrinology 123: 1511–1519
21. Cullinan-Bone K, Koos RD (1993) Vascular endothelial growth factor/vascular permeability factor expression in the rat uterus: rapid stimulation by estrogen correlates with estrogen-induced increases in uterine capillary permeability and growth. Endocrinology 133: 829–837

22. Shmeiki D, Itin A, Neufeld G, et al (1993) Patterns of expression of vascular endothelial growth factor (VEGF) and VEGF receptors in mice suggest a role in hormonally regulated angiogenesis. J Clin Invest 91: 2235–2243
23. Haining RFB, et al (1991) Identification of mRNA for epidermal growth factor and transforming growth factor-α present in low copy number in human endometrium and decidua using reverse transcriptase-polymerase chain reactions. J Mol Endocrinol 6: 207–214
24. Ferriani R, Charnock-Jones DS, Prentice A, et al (1993) Immunohistochemical localization of acidic and basic fibroblast growth factors in normal human endometrium and endometriosis and the detection of their mRNA by polymerase chain reaction. Hum Reprod 8: 11–16
25. Reynolds K, Farzanah F, Collins WP, et al (1994) Correlation of ovarian malignancy with expression of platelet-derived endothelial cell growth factor. J Natl Cancer Inst 86: 1234–1238
26. Jain RK (1988) Determinants of tumor blood flow. A review. Cancer Res 48: 2641–2658
27. Folkman J, Watson K, Ingbar D, Hanahan D (1989) Induction of angiogenesis during the transition from hyperplasia to neoplasia. Nature 339: 58–61
28. Horak ER, Leek R, Klenk N, et al (1992) Quantitative angiogenesis assessed by anti-PECAM (platelet/endothelial cell adhesion molecule) antibodies; correlation with node metastasis and survival in breast cancer. Lancet 340: 1120–1124
29. Eda H, Fujimoto K, Watanabe S-I, et al (1993) Cytokines induce thymidine phosphorylase expression in tumor cells and make them more susceptible to 5'-deoxy-5-fluorouridine. Cancer Chemother Pharmacol 32(5): 333–338

Vascular Anatomy of the Pelvis

G.J. Burton

Introduction

The female internal genitalia derive their blood supply from two principal sources, the uterine and ovarian arteries. The terminal parts of these two vessels anastomose within the broad ligament, and consequently a vascular arcade is established that extends from the cervix to the ovary (Fig. 1). Determining the exact area of distribution of each artery is therefore difficult, but on the basis of in vivo radiographic studies, Borell and Fernström [3] concluded that in the majority of cases the uterine artery contributes the main supply to the medial half of the ovary and the medial two thirds of the fallopian tube in addition to supplying the uterus. The authors stressed, however, that considerable individual variation exists, and in extreme cases either artery may supply the entire uterus and tube. The possibility of such variations should therefore be borne in mind when reading the following account.

Uterine Artery

Origin

Details of the disposition of the major pelvic vessels are available in most of the standard anatomical texts. Opposite the sacro-iliac joint the common iliac artery bifurcates and gives rise to the internal and external iliac arteries. Whilst the former continues around the pelvic brim, the latter passes inferiorly and posteriorly into the pelvis. After approximately 2 cm, the internal iliac artery reaches the superior margin of the greater sciatic notch. At this point it divides into an anterior division, principally distributed to the pelvic viscera, and a posterior division which supplies the surrounding striated musculature.

In the female the uterine artery is the first and largest branch of the anterior division. From its origin the artery runs inferiorly along the lateral wall of the pelvis, across the greater sciatic notch in the posterior part of the ovarian fossa. It is accompanied on its medial side by the ureter, but after approximately 3 cm the artery turns abruptly medially and to a lesser extent anteriorly. This change in direction takes the uterine artery across the anterior surface of the ureter and into the broad ligament at the level of the cardinal ligament. As it crosses the ureter the artery often gives off a small ureteric branch. After running horizontally for 1–2 cm, the uterine artery reaches first the lateral vaginal fornix and then the wall of the uterus. The main vessel turns sharply superiorly at this point towards the utero-tubual junction, whilst a much smaller branch continues on to supply the cervix and upper part of the vagina (Fig. 1). Free anastomoses exist between these vaginal branches of the uterine artery and terminal branches of the true vaginal artery. The latter is also a branch of the anterior division of the internal iliac artery, branching off just distal to the uterine artery either as a single trunk or as a series of two or three parallel arteries. From these anastomoses, two median longitudinal vessels arise, the azygos arteries of the vagina. One runs inferiorly along the anterior surface of the vagina, the other along the posterior surface.

The main continuation of the uterine artery passes within the broad ligament along the lateral wall of the uterus towards the utero-tubual junction. It terminates by dividing into three branches: a recurrent branch which is directed towards the fundus of the uterus, a branch that runs parallel and immediately inferior to the medial part of the fallopian tube and a branch which passes to the hilus of the ovary. The latter two vessels anastomose with their counterpart branches of the ovarian artery, so forming the vascular arcade mentioned previously. Borell and Fernström [3] were unable to distinguish between the tubal and ovarian branches during their radiographic studies and so considered the presence of either to represent an adnexal branch of the uterine artery. They reported finding a significant adnexal branch (of approximately 1 mm in diameter) in 11 out of 18 normal subjects. In contrast, they found one to be present in all nine cases of either acute or chronic salpingitis. This may reflect the fact that in pathological conditions the vessels can dilate, and that in doing so they become easier to detect radiographically.

During its course through the broad ligament, the uterine artery is highly convoluted. It is generally accepted that this tortuosity allows the vessel to accommodate the enormous enlargement of the uterus that takes place during pregnancy, but it is intriguing that this adaptation should be present even in the nulliparous state. At frequent intervals along its course, the artery gives off medial branches, which immediately penetrate the substance of the uterine wall. The fate of these was illustrated clearly by Farrer-Brown et al. [5] by means of a combination of vascular injection and microradiography of operative specimens. Each branch divides into an anterior and a posterior arcuate artery, which run circumferentially around the uterine wall. Terminal branches of the left and right vessels anastomose freely across the midline. The arcuate arteries lie at the level of the junction between the outer and middle thirds of the myometrium and give rise to a subserosal arterial plexus and a capillary plexus surrounding the smooth muscle fibres. They also give rise to a series of radial arteries which pass centripetally through the deeper layers of the myometrium to supply the endometrium. These branches are of two types: straight arteries which branch directly on reaching the endometrium and supply the stratum basalis, and spiral arteries which, as their name suggests, are highly tortuous and penetrate the stratum spongiosum and stratum compactum (Fig. 2). Of the two types, the straight arteries are present

a'
a'
a'
a'
c
c
c
c'
b'
d
b
O.A.
e
U.A.
f
g
g
g
h
h

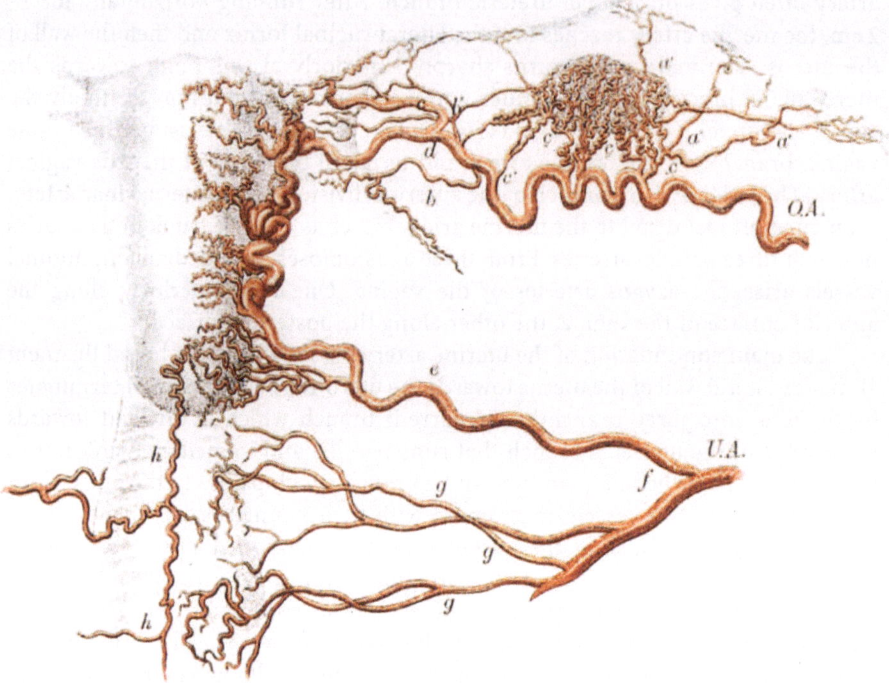

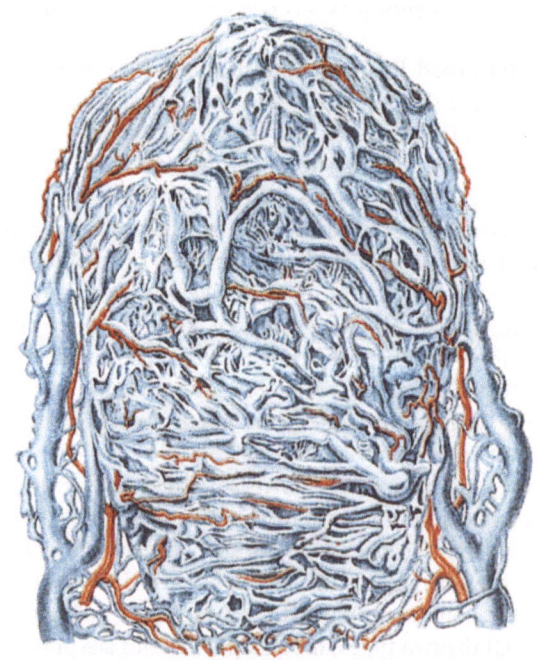

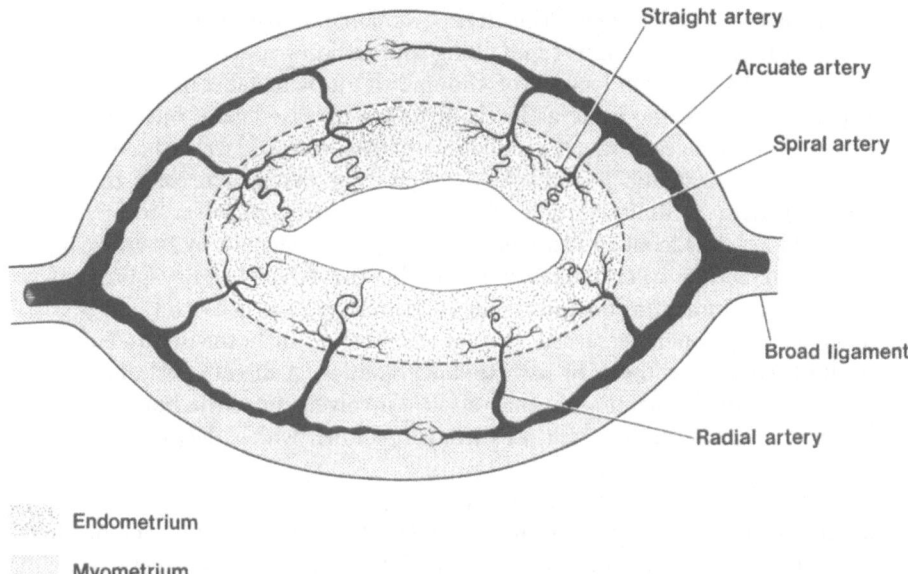

Endometrium

Myometrium

Fig. 2. Transverse section of the uterus. The arcuate arteries lie at the junction between the outer one third and the inner two thirds of the myometrium. Only the spiral arteries undergo changes during the menstrual cycle

at a higher density, but in general the endometrium appears less vascularised than the myometrium.

Anatomical Changes During the Cycle

Significant changes occur in the vasculature during the menstrual cycle, but these are restricted exclusively to the spiral arteries of the endometrium. The foundations of our knowledge were laid by the pioneering work of Bartelmaz [1] on humans, and Markee [10] on the rhesus monkey. Their accounts were integrated and updated in the review of menstruation by Shaw and Roche [12]. During the follicular phase of the cycle, the endometrium thickens as a result of mitotic proliferation of the stromal cells and the spiral arteries under the influence of

---

Fig. 1. The arterial supply and venous drainage of the uterus as revealed by corrosion casting. The ovarian artery (*OA*) follows a tortuous course and gives off branches to the ampullary (*a'*) and isthmic (*b'*) regions of the fallopian tube, as well as branches to the ovary (*c'*). Shortly before anastomosing with the uterine artery (*d*), it provides a small supply to the round ligament (*b*). The uterine artery (*e*) supplies the cervix and then ascends along the side of the uterus within the broad ligament. Several vaginal arteries (*g*) may arise from the internal iliac artery (*f*), and in association with the cervical branches of the uterine artery they form the anterior and posterior azygos arteries of the vagina (*h*). From [8]

increasing levels of oestrogen. The arteries remain of narrow calibre, however, for Farrer-Brown et al. [5] observed no filling with radio-opaque medium beyond the statum basalis. A second phase of endometrial growth takes place during the secretory phase of the cycle as levels of oestrogen rise again, but this time in tandem with progesterone. Vasodilation of the spiral arteries occurs and is linked with a dramatic increase in their permeability, which leads to marked stromal oedema. Administration of exogenous oestrogen causes an increase in uterine blood flow in all species studied so far [7] (see chapter by Bourne et al. on "Ovulation and the Periovulatory Follicle"). The effect begins approximately 30 min after administration and reaches maximal levels after 1–4 h [7]. It is possibly mediated through decreased levels of norepinephrine in the uterus, either as a result of reduced synthesis or increased degradation. A direct effect of oestrogen on smooth muscle membranes may also be involved, since the hormone is still active in animals treated with 6-hydroxydopamine, which destroys adrenergic nerves.

Towards the end of the secretory phase, the spiral arteries show maximal development and visibly reach the endometrial surface, turning back on themselves to form small arcades. Regression of the corpus luteum results in falling levels of oestrogen, however, and consequently the increase in vessel permeability is reversed. Resorption of the oedema fluid leads to shrinkage of the endometrium, particularly in the stratum spongiosum. There is also a decline in the mitotic index of the stromal and glandular cells, whereas the spiral arteries may continue to proliferate until 36 h prior to the menses. The net effect of lengthening vessels in a contracting endometrium is that the spiral arteries become even more tightly coiled. This increased tortuosity most likely impedes blood flow, an effect exacerbated by medial constriction in response to oestrogen withdrawal. Stasis gradually occurs in the distal microvasculature, and tissue hypoxia is generally considered to be the direct cause of degenerative changes seen within the superficial endometrium. An acute inflammatory response ensues, with the generation of vasoactive amines. These are thought to cause the particularly intense constriction of the spiral arteries that has been reported to precede the onset of menstrual bleeding, which is followed by an equally abrupt vasodilation of individual vessels. The resumption of flow in the ischaemically damaged distal segments of the vessels leads to diapedesis of erythrocytes into the stromal tissue and sloughing of the superficial layers of the endometrium.

Ovarian Artery

The left and right ovarian arteries arise from the anterior surface of the aorta just below the origin of the renal arteries at the level of the second lumbar vertebra. On each side, the artery then runs inferiorly and slightly laterally across the surface of the psoas major muscle to reach the pelvic brim. At this point it crosses the anterior surface of the ureter at an acute angle, passing from medial to lateral. The artery then enters the pelvis anterior to the internal iliac vessels and passes via the suspensory ligament of the ovary into the broad ligament. Close to the ovary the main artery divides into several unequal branches.

The largest division enters the mesovarium and follows a highly tortuous course towards the hilus of the ovary. It is closely surrounded by an elaborate venous plexus associated with the ovarian vein, and there is extensive and intimate contact between the two sets of vessel walls [2]. In many species this arrangement is believed to permit countercurrent exchange of leuteolytic prostaglandins from the uterine to the ovarian circulation [4]. In the human female, leuteolysis is not achieved in this manner, but the same anatomical arrangement may serve to increase the levels of chorionic gonadotrophin in the ovary during the immediate post-implantation period. At the hilus of the ovary, the main ovarian artery anastomoses with the ovarian branch of the uterine artery as previously mentioned (Fig. 1). The combined vessel gives off a number of branches which pass into the medullary region of the gland. These branches also have a tight spiral configuration, although the degree of tortuosity decreases after the menopause. It is widely believed that this configuration again allows the vessels to accommodate the changing size of the organ during the various phases of the menstrual cycle, but equalisation of blood flows and reduction in blood pressure have also been suggested as reasons [11]. Studies of corrosion casts of the vasculature have revealed that during follicular growth there are many coiled arteries, but after ovulation these undergo progressive extension, eventually uncoiling and becoming sinuous [9]. The terminal branches of these vessels also undergo extensive modifications, forming a capillary plexus within the theca interna during folliculogenesis and then invading the granulosa of the corpus luteum.

A second smaller branch of the ovarian artery runs medially in the broad ligament, parallel and just inferior to the fallopian tube. It ends by anastomosing with the tubal branch of the uterine artery and forms a vascular arcade which supplies numerous fine branches to the tube.

A third branch is directed towards the infundibular part of the fallopian tube, and lastly a very minor branch passes along the round ligament of the uterus towards the deep inguinal ring.

Venous Drainage

In general the venous drainage of the internal genitalia satellites the arterial supply. Within the endometrium there are numerous veins, and these tend to run parallel to the glandular columns [6]. By comparison the inner half of the myometrium is relatively avascular, and a second dense network is found just below the serosal surface. Veins emerging from this form an extensive uterine plexus within the broad ligament, which communicates freely with the ovarian and vaginal plexuses. Two uterine veins usually drain the uterine plexus on each side. These arise at the level of the cardinal ligaments and join the corresponding internal iliac vein. The vaginal plexus is particularly well developed around the lower portion and is commonly drained by a single vein which is also a tributary of the internal iliac vein. The plexus is also in free communication with the rectal and vesical plexuses.

The veins emerging at the hilus of the ovary form an elaborate plexus, the pampiniform plexus. As previously mentioned these vessels are in extensive and intimate contact with the ovarian artery. Towards the lateral margin of the broad ligament, the plexus converges to give rise to two ovarian veins which subsequently unite. The veins accompany the ovarian artery and drain into the inferior vena cava on the right and the renal vein on the left. Valves may occasionally be present within the ovarian veins.

Bladder Vascularisation

The main blood supply to the bladder is provided by the superior and inferior vesical arteries. The former represents the still patent part of the foetal umbilical artery and arises from the anterior division of the internal iliac artery either close to or in common with the uterine artery. It follows a short course inferio-medially and is distributed to the upper parts of the bladder. The inferior vesical is a later branch of the anterior division of the internal iliac artery, branching off opposite the greater sciatic notch. It may share a joint origin with the middle rectal artery and runs along the surface of the levator ani muscle to supply the lower parts of the organ. Finally, there may be a small contribution from the vaginal arteries to the fundic region.

Venous drainage takes place by way of a rich vesical plexus surrounding the lower part of the organ. From this plexus a single vesical vein usually emerges and drains into the internal iliac vein.

References

1. Bartelmaz GW (1933) Histological studies on the menstruating mucous membrane of the human uterus. Contr Embryol 24: 141–186
2. Bendz A (1982) On the extensive contact between veins and arteries in the human ovarian pedicle. Acta Physiol Scand 115: 179–182
3. Borell U, Fernström I (1953) The adnexal branches of the uterine artery. An arteriographic study in human subjects. Acta Radiol 40: 561–582
4. Einer-Jensen N (1988) Countercurrent transfer in the ovarian pedicle and its physiological implications. Oxf Rev Reprod Biol 10: 348–381
5. Farrer-Brown G, Beilby JOW, Tarbit MH (1970a) The blood supply of the uterus. 1. Arterial vasculature. J Obstet Gynaecol Br Commonw 77: 673–681
6. Farrer-Brown G, Beilby JOW, Tarbit MH (1970b) The blood supply of the uterus. 2. Venous pattern. J Obstet Gynaecol Br Commonw 77: 682–689
7. Ford SP (1989) Factors controlling uterine blood flow during estrous and early pregnancy. In: Rosenfield CR (ed) The uterine circulation. Perinatology, New York, pp 113–134
8. Hyrtl J (1873) Die Corrosions – Anatomie und ihre Ergebnisse. Braunmüller, Vienna
9. Kessel RG, Kardon RH (1979) Tissues and organs: a text-atlas of scanning electron microscopy. Freeman, San Francisco

10. Markee JE (1940) Menstruation in intraocular endometrial transplants in the rhesus monkey. Contr Embryol 28: 221–308
11. Reynolds SRM (1973) Blood and lymph vascular systems of the ovary. In: Greep RO, Astwood EB (eds) Handbook of physiology, vol 7/2. American Physiological Society, Bethesda, pp 261–316
12. Shaw ST Jr, Roche PC (1980) Menstruation. Oxf Rev Reprod Biol 2: 41–96

The Human Heart – Development of Form and Function

G. Moscoso

Introduction

Diagnosis in the field of foetal medicine is fast improving its specificity and sensitivity with the help of rapid advances in ultrasound and biomolecular technology. The immediate results are on the one hand a more accurate diagnosis and on the other a greater demand for accurate data on normal parameters of development of form and function at ever earlier stages of pregnancy.

This chapter highlights some aspects of normal cardiovascular development at organ, cell and molecular levels and uses some abnormal conditions to postulate the pathological basis of dysfunction.

Development of Form

In humans, the heart is among the first organs to develop and to function in early embryonic life. Studies of the anatomical changes occurring during morphogenesis in this complex four-chamber organ have been greatly improved by the combined use of microdissection and scanning electron microscopy [27, 30].

During the third week of gestation, just before the formation of the first two to three somites (Streeter's stage VIII), beneath the cephalic end of the embryonic plate, a plexus of primitive vessels forms on either side of the midline. Similar findings have been documented in some animal models by Linask et al. [21, 22]. As the first somites differentiate during the 19th/20th day (Streeter's stage IX), the fast developing vascular plexus forms two larger, paired vessels, which fuse in the midline to form the primitive cardiac tube by the 20th/22nd day of gestation (Streeter's stage XI).

Towards the 24th day (Streeter's stage XI), the primitive cardiac tube bends forwards, forming a loop which gradually rotates to the right. This accelerated growth is, in part, explained by cell differentiation and intercellular matrix generation [25]. By the 28th–29th day (Streeter's stage XII), following the direction of blood flow, an inlet, a transverse and outlet segments can be recognized (Fig. 1).

Internally, the cardiac tube is lined by primitive endocardial cells and its thick walls are made up of cardiac jelly, found to be a locally extended form of basement membrane secreted by the outer myocardial layer of the heart tube [20]. Gradually, the cardiac jelly becomes populated by migrating cells from the primitive endocar-

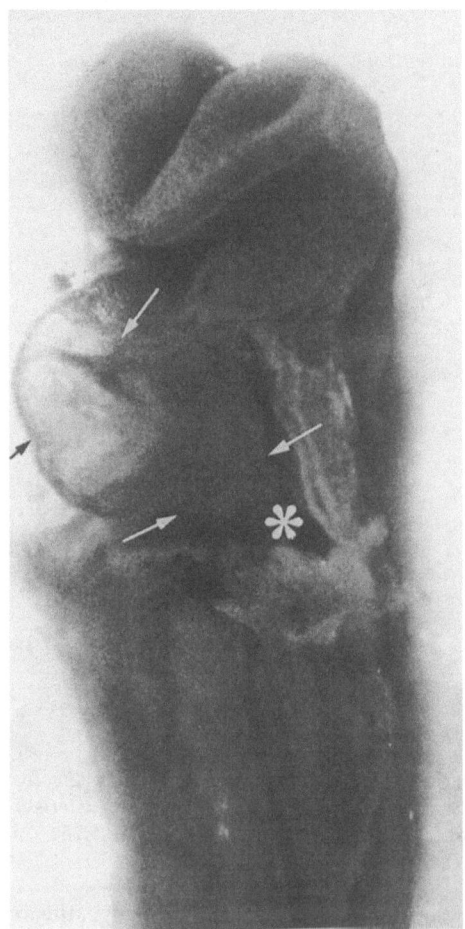

Fig. 1. Human embryo at 24 days of gestation (Streeter's stage XI). A left oblique view shows the inlet portion of the cardiac loop. There are two small constrictions at this level (*arrows*). The *asterisk* marks the developing pericardial space

dium (Fig. 2). Migration of cells is induced by specific agents, generated in selected segments of the cardiac tube, i.e. those where the atrio-ventricular cushions differentiate [26, 32]. Using radioisotope labelling methods, the biochemical composition of the cardiac jelly has been shown to contain glycosaminoglycans, collagen and other glycoproteins [16, 23, 24].

At 32 days (Streeter's stage XV), both atria, the developing left and right ventricles and the truncus arteriosus can be identified on external examination (Fig. 3).

Internally, the valves of the sinus venosus and the septum primum are already present. Thus a primitive right and left atria can be recognized. Caudal to the septum primum, though adjacent to it, are the dorsal and ventral atrio-ventricular cushions. They appear opposite to each other, as two separate wedge-shaped eminences. More importantly, they delineate the atrio-ventricular boundaries and will contribute to the differentiation of the atrio-ventricular valvular apparatus

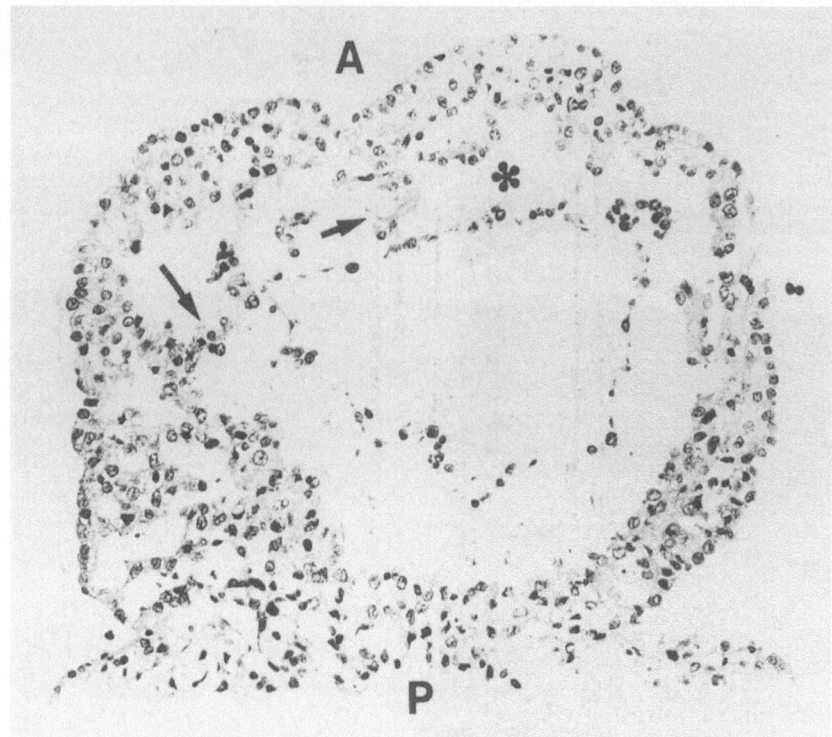

Fig. 2. Cephalic view of the inlet section of the cardiac loop, cut in a transverse plane, from a human embryo at 22 days of gestation (Streeter's stage XI). The cardiac jelly (*asterisk*) is populated by migrating cells (*arrows*). Frontal (*A*) and dorsal (*P*) planes. H&E, ×250

(Fig. 4). The emerging interventricular septum resembles a shallow ridge, the axis of which is perpendicular to the atrioventricular cushions. The unique topological distribution of the unfused atrio-ventricular cushions above and the developing interventricular septum below determine the foramen interventriculare primum, a bridging space communicating between the primitive right and left ventricular chambers (Fig. 4).

In the conotruncal region at the level of the outlet segment of the cardiac loop, two unfused ridges can be observed running along the longer axis of the conotruncus. These ridges appear broad, shallow and less well defined when observed at their proximal and distal ends. In contrast, they become somewhat taller and therefore better defined in their mid-portion (Fig. 4).

Fusion of the atrio-ventricular cushions and truncal ridges occurs during the 32nd–38th day of gestation (Streeter's stage XVI) and a clear atrio-ventricular continuity, guarded by the developing atrio-ventricular valves, can be observed. Interestingly, the morphological markers which help in differentiating a right from a left ventricle are not apparent as this stage.

At 42 days of gestation, the foramen interventriculare secundum remains

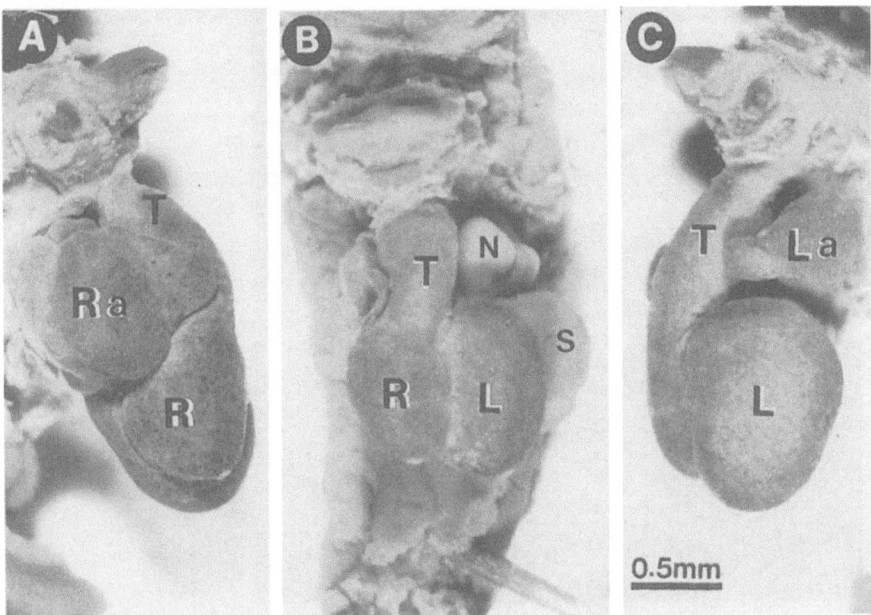

Fig. 3A–C. Heart from a human embryo at 32 days of gestation. Both atria (*Ra, La*) and ventricles (*R, L*) are clearly visible. Note the presence of the truncus arteriosus (*T*). *N,* Left lung; *S,* stomach **A** Right view. **B** Frontal view. **C** Left view

patent. Its roof is formed by the overriding subaortic infundibulum, the anterior and inferior margins by the ridge of the interventricular septum and the posterior margin by the fused atrio-ventricular cushions. Their right tubercles are clearly visible on the septal aspect of the right ventricle. At this stage, there is no evidence of a septal leaflet of the tricuspid valve. The right ventricular outflow tract is well defined, and the developing semilunar cusps of both the aortic and pulmonary valves show an even and simultaneous process of differentiation. From the earliest stages there is a haemodynamic connection or blood flow "streaming" towards the aorta from the left ventricle, although at this point of organogenesis the aorta is not anatomically connected to the left ventricle. Preferential streaming is presumably achieved, in part, with the help of the parietal leaflet of the tricuspid valve which, during early systole, occludes the foramen interventriculare as well as the inlet portion of the right ventricle (Fig. 5). Thus, blood would "stream" into the aorta from the left ventricle only.

Fusion of the conotruncal ridges divides the truncus arteriosus into the ascending aorta and the main pulmonary artery and modulates the formation of the right and left ventricular outflow tracts. From the outset, both great arteries maintain a typical spatial relationship with one another, although at this stage the aorta is structurally related to the right ventricle. When observed from a cephalic view, the pulmonary trunk is connected to the developing right ventricle; it is anterior and slightly to the right of the ascending aorta. Conversely, the ascending aorta is

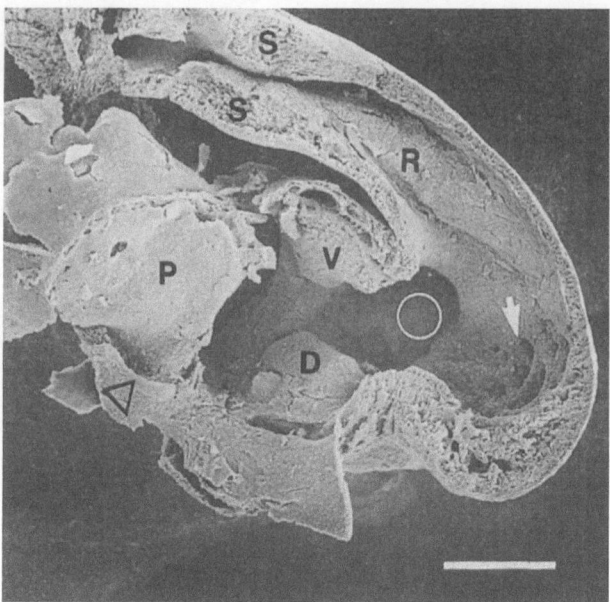

Fig. 4. Human embryonic heart at 32 days of gestation (Streeter's stage XV). The right lateral wall of both the right atrium and right ventricle together with that of the conotruncus have been removed. The septum primum (*P*) and the developing valve of the sinus venosus (*arrowhead*) are at a distance from the unfused ventral (*V*) and dorsal (*D*) atrio-ventricular cushions. The foramen interventriculare primum is patent (*circle*). Its lower margin is formed by the developing interventricular septum. Note the left anterolateral ridge (*R*). At the distal margins of the truncus arteriosus are the valve swellings (*S*) of the putative aorta and pulmonary trunk. The *arrow* points to the developing embryonic trabeculae in the apical region of the right ventricle. *Scale bar*, 250 μm. SEM, ×56

posterior to the pulmonary trunk and slightly to the left. Internally, the pulmonary trunk is fully connected to the right ventricular outflow tract, whereas the aorta overrides the ventricular septum, therefore indicating that it is already partly committed to the left ventricle; the right lateral aspect of the subaortic infundibulum is between the developing crista supraventricularis anteriorly and the anterior leaflet of the tricuspid valve posteriorly, all right ventricular structures (Fig. 6). This brief but complex spatial relationship, ignored until recently, became apparent when investigating the embryonic human heart using the scanning electron microscope.

As cardiac morphogenesis continues, the aorta looses its continuity with the right ventricle, whilst, for a short period of time, the subaortic infundibulum overrides the interventricular septum, before connecting to the left ventricle. Meanwhile, the interventricular septum has grown and both ventricular chambers have increased in volume and show well-developed embryonic trabeculae.

Delamination of the atrio-ventricular valve leaflets follow a predictable pat-

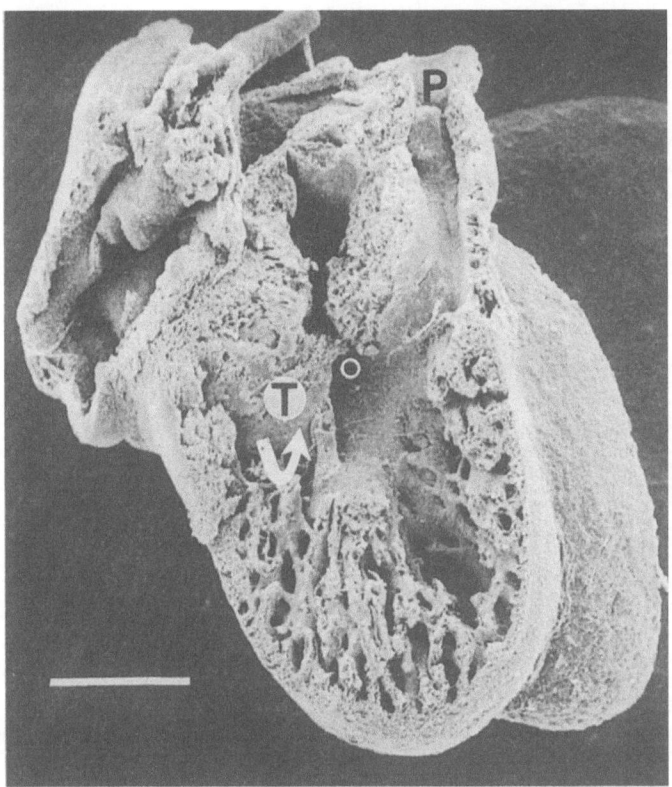

Fig. 5. Human embryonic heart at 42 days of gestation. The topology of the various ventricular components resemble that observed in early systole. During early ventricular contraction, the parietal leaflet of the tricuspid valve (*T*) has approximated (*arrow*) and therefore partly occluded the foramen interventriculare (*O*), favouring a left ventricle to aortic blood flow. *Scale bar*, 250 µm. SEM, ×69

tern. The anterior leaflet of the tricuspid valve and both the anterolateral and posteromedial leaflets of the mitral valve appear shortly after fusion of the atrio-ventricular cushions and conotruncal ridges. However, delamination of the septal leaflet of the tricuspid valve takes place after closure of the foramen interventriculare tertium during the seventh to eighth week of gestation (Fig. 7).

At 32 days of gestation (Streeter's stage XV), embryonic trabeculae emerge as shallow ridges in the apical endocardial region of the primitive ventricles (Fig. 4). At 42 days (Streeter's stage XVII), well-developed embryonic trabeculae cross the ventricular chambers, creating a number of ventricular sinuses. Such a spatial distribution gives a sponge-like appearance to the internal relief of both ventricles. Definitive trabeculae form and run parallel to the ventricular walls. They appear towards the 40th day of gestation, first at the level of the atrio-ventricular junction in the free walls of both ventricles and develop towards the apex. Furthermore, they do not cross the ventricular chambers. As definitive trabeculae grow and

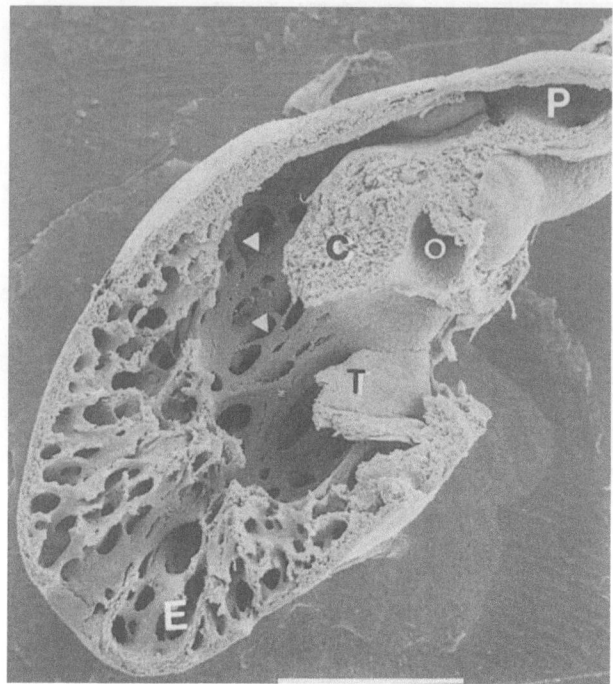

Fig. 6. Parietal aspect of a human right ventricle at 42 days of gestation, before closure of the foramen interventriculare. The subaortic infundibulum (*O*) is directly related to the crista supraventricularis (*C*) and the anterior leaflet of the tricuspid valve (*T*). The pulmonary trunk (*P*) is connected to the right ventricular outflow tract. Note the embryonic trabeculae (*E*). Some definitive trabeculae are present (*arrowheads*). *Scale bar*, 500 µm. SEM, ×65

proliferate, the embryonic trabeculae appear to be displaced to the apical region of the ventricles. Definitive trabeculae are observed during the 40th day of gestation and they predominate in the free walls of both ventricles by the seventh week of gestation (Fig. 6). At 10 weeks, there are fewer embryonic trabeculae confined to the apical region and these gradually become thinner, divide and their loose ends are reabsorbed (Fig. 8). This remodelling process is accomplished without the intervention of macrophages or inflammatory cells in the immediate interstitium. It should be remembered that programmed cell death is also a powerful morphogenetic mechanism, very much expressed during organogenesis [29].

Towards the end of the sixth week of gestation (Streeter's stage XVIII), the aorta is anatomically connected to the left ventricle. The foramen interventriculare tertium, measuring about 80 µm in its largest diameter, closes in a right to left interventricular direction. A "dimple" less than 40 µm in diameter is left briefly at the site of closure on the endocardial surface of the left ventricle. Closure of the foramen interventriculare tertium completes the anatomical structure for a parallel-circuit mode of circulation, typical in foetal life.

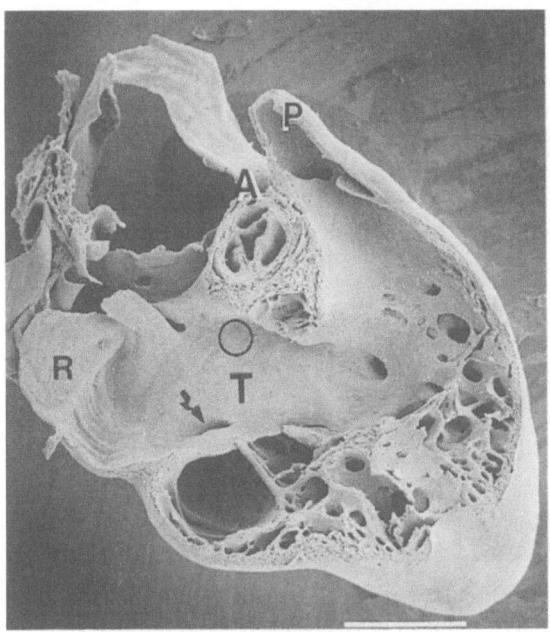

Fig. 7. Septal aspect of the right ventricle of a human heart at 8 weeks of gestation. Delamination of the septal leaflet of the tricuspid valve (*T*) is taking place. A cleft (*black arrow*) marks the posterior margin of the septal leaflet. There are no clefts delineating the anterior margins in the region adjacent to the crista supraventricularis. Note the endocardial continuity at this level (*open circle*). No tension apparatus is present. *R*, Right atrium; *A*, aortic valve; *P*, pulmonary trunk, *Scale bar*, 500 μm. SEM, ×40

Differentiation of the tension apparatus and papillary muscles takes place after the eighth week of gestation. It occurs at about the same pace in both atrioventricular valves. In contrast, the development of the ventricular mass is different in right and left ventricles. A predominant ventricular mass and a thicker free wall are already apparent in the left ventricle before closure of the foramen interventriculare. Furthermore, the combined weight of both ventricles increases more than threefold, from 50 mg at 9 weeks to over 150 mg at 14 weeks. The factors responsible for such selective differential growth between the ventricles are not known. However, it is of interest that, after the tenth week of gestation, the placental circulation enters a phase of rapid growth [15]. Thus, foetal growth and a rapidly enlarging placental vascular bed may account, in part, for the selective increase in left ventricular wall thickness.

During the eighth to ninth week of gestation, differentiation of the membranous portion of the ventricular septum starts, largely from residual atrio-ventricular cushion tissue. Simultaneously, the aortic valve is establishing an ever closer anatomical continuity with the anterolateral leaflet of the mitral valve. At 11 weeks of gestation, differentiation of the membranous portion of the ventricular septum is well under way. Its completion marks the end of cardiac organogenesis. At this

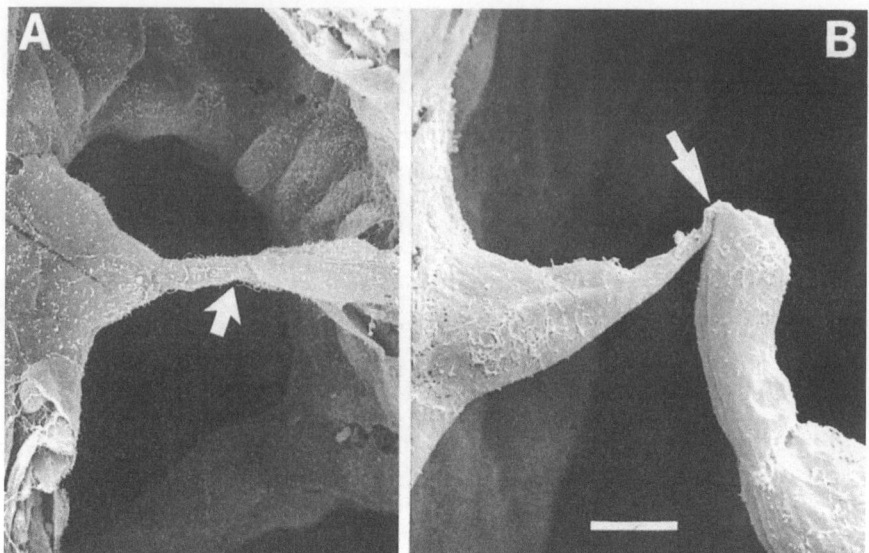

Fig. 8. A One-cell thick embryonic trabecula (*arrow*). SEM, ×1300. **B** Following separation, two embryonic trabecula are united by a thread of residual cytoplasm (*arrow*). *Scale bar,* 5 μm. SEM, ×3000

point, the external and internal morphology of the human heart closely resembles that observed later in gestation or after birth.

Genetic and Molecular Basis of Morphogenesis

It has been accepted that maternally inherited information regulates the earliest stages of embryonic development in some mammalian species [7]. In humans, gene expression occurs during the pre-implantation period between the fourth and eighth cell stages [4].

Homeobox genes encode a class of regulatory proteins which participate in the development of form [1, 9, 10]. In the developing chick heart, expression of homeobox genes *Msx-1* (*hox-7*) has been observed in a variety of cells undergoing transformation in the atrio-ventricular and outflow tract regions, and it is thought they may play a role in septation and valve formation. In contrast, *Msx-2* (*Hox-8*) is expressed in a region corresponding to the conducting system of the heart [5].

Gene expression and the resulting post-translational molecules in charge of modulating cardiogenesis determine patterns of cell migration to pre-determined regions of the heart by following extracelluar biochemical cues [21, 22]. Furthermore, it has been shown that neural cell adhesion molecules (N-CAM) have been implicated in modulating the process of morphogenesis in a variety of organ systems (see [8] for review). We have demonstrated that there is a greater N-CAM expression in the cardiac muscle early in foetal life. Interestingly, due to a process of down-regulation, N-CAM expression is confined, by the end of pregnancy, to nerve fibres and ganglion cells innervating the heart. More importantly, we have observed that there is a significant re-expression of N-CAM in pathological conditions such as cardiac hypertrophy or after heart transplant [11]. This suggests that, during hypertrophy or during tissue repair and regeneration following transplant, the heart activates a selected set of genes that once were used during morphogenesis. It has been known for some time that migration of cells from the neural crest participate in the development of the outflow tract and in the post-ganglionic cardiac innervation [17]. This is an extensive subject, beyond the scope of this chapter, and therefore will not be addressed further here.

Cardiogenesis in the human does not mean the exclusive development of contractile cardiac muscle and valvular components correctly assembled [2]. There is also a simultaneous process of specific cytochemical differentiation during cardiac morphogenesis as gestation approaches term. Atrial natriuretic peptide (ANP) can be identified in both atria and ventricles as early as 7 weeks of gestation [31, 33, 35], and it has been considered as an important regulator of the circulatory volume. Wilhelm et al. [36] have shown abnormally high levels of ANP in the amniotic fluid of foetuses affected by hydrops or with cardiovascular malformations. Therefore, cytochemical cell differentiation for ANP synthesis and other active peptides such as endothelin or nitric oxides occurs parallel to the development of form. More importantly, they follow a pattern of expression of their own.

Form and Function

In the heart, the development of form is inextricably linked to the development of function. At present, in spite of significant advances in foetal echocardiography and the recently improved technology applied to colour Doppler ultrasound, the precise regulatory mechanisms determining normal foetal blood flow are yet to be defined. Nonetheless, the assessment of blood velocity profiles is proving to be an excellent tool for identifying abnormal pregnancies. Furthermore, the study of venous blood flow through the ductus venosus using colour Doppler ultrasound has prompted a review of the anatomy of a subdiaphragmatic venous vestibulum ignored until now which, it appears, plays an active role in modulating blood flow into the left atrium [13]. Furthermore, the application of colour Doppler ultrasound is helping us to understand the haemodynamic events of venous blood flow occurring between the sinus venosus and the left atrium. It is now accepted that due to "preferential streaming", oxygenated blood carried by the ductus venosus enters the left atrium during atrial diastole, by-passing the right atrium [19]. More importantly, blood velocity in the inferior vena cava slows down, whilst that in the ductus venous accelerates during atrial systole [18]. The latter therefore provides, a "head" of oxygenated blood waiting at the door of the foramen ovale to enter the left atrium during the next diastole when atrial filling occurs. If this is true, the left atrium should receive a continuous stream of oxygenated blood, whilst the right atrium would receive an intermittent spill-over of oxygenated blood. The ductus venosus may not be the only temporary vascular segment playing an important haemodynamic role during foetal life. The venous return from the upper segment of the body ending up in the superior vena cava may also be a box full of haemodynamic surprises. It has been shown that foetuses affected by trisomy 21 present with increased nuchal no leave in as translucency thickness during the second trimester of pregnancy [3]. Furthermore, the degree of this translucency was increased when cardiovascular malformations were present. Recently, it was demonstrated that an increased nuchal translucency of 3 mm or more is a useful marker for chromosomal abnormalities in first-trimester foetuses [28]. We have examined the cardiovascular system of trisomy-affected foetuses who presented during the first trimester with a nuchal translucency of 3 mm or more and found that there is up to an 83% incidence of complex cardiac defects in trisomy 21-affected cases (Fig. 9). In addition, all six cases of trisomy 18 and the two cases of trisomy 13 also presented with cardiac malformations ranging from ventricular septal defects in the trisomy 18 group to atrio-ventricular septal defects or truncus arteriosus in the group affected by trisomy 13. More importantly, one case of Klinefelter's syndrome and one of a tetraploidy also presented with increased nuchal translucency thickness during the first trimester. Therefore, it is becoming

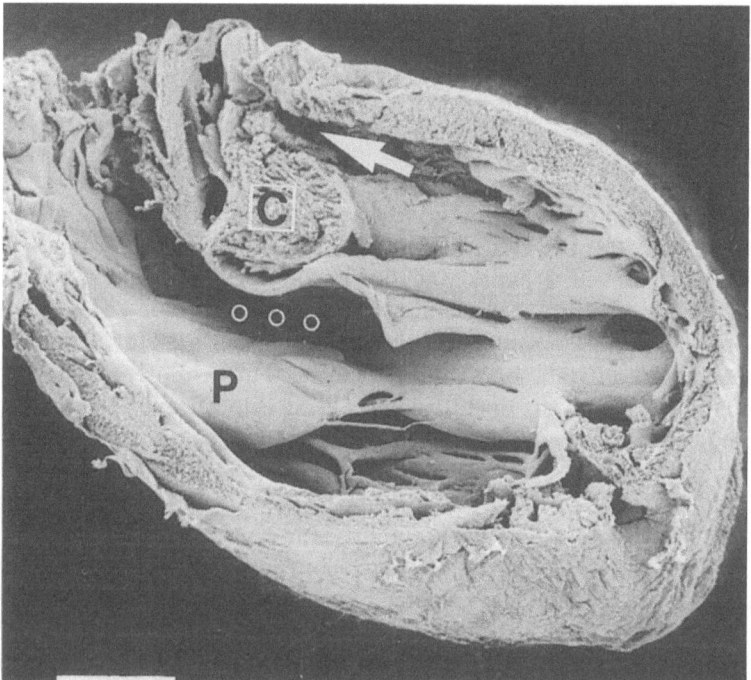

Fig. 9. The right septal aspect of a heart from a trisomy 21 patient presenting with a nuchal translucency of 5 mm at 11 weeks of gestation. Note the atrio-ventricular septal defect (*OOO*) and the dilated right ventricular chamber. *P*, Posterior common atrioventricular valve; *C*, crista supraventricularis. The *arrow* shows the right ventricular outflow tract. *Scale bar*, 500 μm. SEM, ×69

apparent that a direct relationship exists between the degree of nuchal translucency and the severity of the cardiovascular malformation in most of the cases with abnormal karyotype. However, within the group of trisomy 21, there were two cases with a nuchal translucency of 3 mm in which no cardiovascular malformation was identified at organ level (Hyatt, Moscoso and Nicolaides, unpublished observations). To date neither the source nor the biochemical composition of the fluid responsible for an increased nuchal translucency thickness have been determined. However, it may represent an early form of cardiac oedema due to an increased venous pressure in the right atrium, transmitted distally through the superior vena cava. Unlike the inferior vena cava–ductus venous system, in which there are thicker walls and a gradient at the ductus venosus level, the veins proximal to the heart including the superior vena cava have relatively thinner walls. Furthermore, in first trimeter foetuses, examination of this venous system after perfusion–fixation shows the superior vena cava and jugular veins well distended, therefore giving the subjective impression that this segment of the venous circulation in the neck could act as a capacitance area, should the pressure in the right atrium increased abnormally (G. Moscoso, personal observations). Moreover, their thin wall structure could also facilitate easy diffusion of oedema fluid into the adjacent tissues, thus increasing the nuchal translucency thickness. Interestingly, in mouse foetal trisomy 13 cases with cardiovascular malformations, dorsal oedema was observed in 6.4% of cases at 13 days, none at 14 days, in 12.5% at 14 days and 8 h, in 31% at 14 days and 16 h and in 56% of cases at 15 days. Surprisingly, a similar type of oedema was observed in 8.2% at 14 days and 16 h and in 5.1% of cases at 16 days in mouse embryos with normal karyotype [34]. Working with the same trisomy 13 foetal mouse model, Hongell et al. [12] have observed small-size foetuses, cleft palate and transitory oedema of the back and neck. In this animal model as in man, the oedema could ultimately be related to leaking jugular lymphatic sacs due in part to the underlying cardiac defects, as was postulated by Clark [6].

It has been established that the development of both form and function in the human heart is intimately related from the earliest stages of cardiogenesis onwards. If a change in form is the result of a force acting over a mass, as novel concepts in molecular cell engineering suggest [14], then assuming that all things are equal "at the beginning", one could be tempted to say that normal molecular form guarantees normal function. This hypothesis remains to be confirmed.

References

1. Balling R, et al (1989) Craniofacial abnormalities induced by ectopic expression of the homeobox gene Hox-1.1 in transgenic mice. Cell 58: 337
2. Barton PJR, Moscoso G, Thompson R (1991) Detection of myosin gene expression in cardiac muscle using probes derived by polymerase chain reaction (PCR). Int J Cardiol 30: 116–118
3. Benacerraf BR, Gelman R, Frigoletto FD (1987) Sonographic identification of second-trimester fetuses with Down's syndrome. N Engl J Med 317: 1371–1376

4. Braude P, Bolton V, Moore S (1988) Human gene expression occurs between the fourth-and-eight-cell syages of preimplantation development. Nature 332: 459–461
5. Chan-Thomas PS, Thompson RP, Robert B, Yacoub MH, Barton PJ (1993) Expression of homebox genes Msx-1 (Hox-7) and Msx-2 (Hox-8) during cardiac development in the chick. Dev Dyn 197: 203–216
6. Clark EB (1984) Neck web and congenital heart defects: a pathogenic association in 45XO Turner's syndrome? Teratology 29: 355–361
7. Davidson EH (1986) Gene activity in early development. Academic, New York
8. Edelman GM (1988) Topobiology. An introduction to molecular embryology. Basic, New York
9. Gaunt SJ, Sharpe PT, Duboule D (1991) Spatially restricted domains of homeo-genes transcripts in mouse embryos: relation to a segmented body plan. Development 104 [Suppl]: 169–179
10. Gehring WJ (1987) Homeo boxes in the study of development. Science 236: 1245
11. Gordon L, Wharton J, Moore SE, et al (1990) Myocardial localization and isoforms of neural cell adhesion molecule (N-CAM) in the developing and transplanted human heart. J Clin Invest 86: 1293–1300
12. Hongell K, Gropp A (1982) Trisomy 13 in the mouse. Teratology 26: 95–104
13. Huisman TWA, Gittemberg-de-Groot AC, Wladimiroff JW (1992) Recognition of a fetal subdiaphragmatic venous vestibulum essential for fetal venous doppler assessment. Pediatr Res 32: 338–341
14. Ingber DE (1993) The riddle of morphogenesis: a question of solution chemistry or molecular cell engineering? Cell 75: 1249–1252
15. Jauniaux E, Burton GJ, Moscoso G, Hustin J (1991) Development of the early human placenta: a morphometric study. Placenta 12: 269–276
16. Johnson R, Manasek FJ, Vinson W, Seyer J (1974) The biochemical and ultrastructural demonstration of collagen during early heart development. Dev Biol 36: 252–271
17. Kirby ML (1988) Role of extracardiac factors in cardiac development. Experientia 44: 944–951
18. Kiserud T, Eik-Nes SH, Blaas H-G, Hellevik LR (1991) Ultrasonographic velocimetry of the fetal ductus venosus. Lancet 338: 1412–1414
19. Kiserud T, Eik-Nes SH, Blaas H-G, Hellevik LR (1992) Foramen ovale: an ultrasonographic study of its relation to the inferior vena cava, ductus venosus and hepatic veins. Ultrasound Obstet Gynecol 2: 389–394
20. Krug EL, Runyan RB, Markwald RR (1985) Protein extracts from early embryonic hearts initiate cardiac endothelial differentiation. Dev Biol 112: 414–426
21. Linask KK, Lash JW (1986) Precardiac cell migration: fibronectin localisation at meso-derm/endoderm interface during directional movement. Dev Biol 114: 87–101
22. Linask KK, Lash JW (1988) A role for fibronectin in the migration of avian precardiac cells: Dose dependent effects of FN antibody. Dev Biol 129: 135–329
23. Manasek FJ, Reid M, Vinson W, Seyer J, Johnson R (1973) Glycosamynoglycan synthesis by the early embryonic chick heart. Dev Biol 35: 332–348
24. Manasek JF (1976) Glycoprotein synthesis and tissue interaction during establishment of the functional embryonic chick heart. J Mol Cell Cardiol 8: 389–402
25. Manasek JF (1981) Determinants of heart shape in early embryos. Fed Proc 40: 2011–2016
26. Mjaatvedt CH, Lepera RC, Markwald RR (1987) Myocardial specificity of initiating endothelial mesenchymal cell transition in embryonic chick heart correlates with a particular distribution of fibronectin. Dev Biol 119: 59–67
27. Moscoso G, Pexieder T (1991) Variations in microscopic anatomy and ultrastructure of human embryonic hearts subjected to three different modes of fixation. Pathol Res Pract 186: 768–774
28. Nicolaides KH, Azar G, Byrne D, Mansur C, Marks K (1992) Fetal nuchal translucency: ultrasound screening for chromosomal defects in first trimester of pregnancy. BMJ 304: 867–869

29. Pexieder T (1975) Cell death in the morphogenesis and teratogenesis of the heart. Advances in anatomy, embryology and cell biology, vol 51, fasc 3. Springer, Berlin Heidelberg New York
30. Pexieder T (1986) Standardized method for study of normal and abnormal cardiac development in chick, rat, mouse and dog. Teratology 33: 91C–92C (abstr)
31. Pucci A, Wharton J, Arbustini E, Moscoso G, Polak JM, et al (1992) Localization of brain and atrial natriuretic peptide in human and porcine heart. Int J Cardiol 34: 237–247
32. Runyan RB, Markwald RR (1983) Invasion of mesenchyme into three-dimensional collagen gels: A regional and temporal analysis of interaction in embryonic heart tissue. Dev Biol 95: 108–114
33. Takemura G, Fujiwara H, Mukoyama M, et al (1991) Expression and distribution of atrial natriuretic peptide in human hypertrophic ventricle of hypertensive hearts and hearts with hypertrophic cardiomyopathy. Circulation 83: 181–190
34. Vuillemin M, Pexieder T, Winking H (1991) Pathogenesis of various forms of double outlet right ventricle in mouse fetal trisomy 13. Int J Cardiol 33: 281–304
35. Wharton J, Anderson RH, Springall D, et al (1988) Localization of atrial natriuretic peptide immunoreactivity in the ventricular myocardium and conduction system of the human fetal and adult heart. Br Heart J 60: 267–274
36. Wilhelm L, Luckhaus J, Gembruch U (1991) Intrauterine fetal ANP levels as an indicator of cardiac overload. Fetal Diag Ther p5 (abstr)

Vascular Features of Gynaecological Neoplasms

H. Fox

Introduction

The vascularity of gynaecological tumours has long been considered as a some-what recondite aspect of oncological biology but has, with the advent of transvaginal colour flow Doppler, now achieved practical importance. It is intended in this brief review to consider the general mechanisms of tumour angiogenesis and control of tumour blood flow together with the clinical significance of gynaecological tumour vascularization.

Angiogenesis

Angiogenesis occurs in a wide range of both physiological and pathological conditions, but in all circumstances follows a stereotyped pattern of sequential steps [8]. New capillaries originate from small venules or other capillaries. One of the first steps in this process is local destruction of the basement membrane of the venule on the side closest to the angiogenic stimulus, possibly because of local secretion of collagenases by stimulated endothelial cells. Endothelial cells then migrate through the gap in the basement membrane and align themselves to form capillary sprouts; endothelial cell mitotic activity is seen in the mid-section of the sprout, but the endothelial cells at the tip of the sprout, whilst continuing to migrate towards the angiogenic stimulus, do not undergo division. A lumen forms within the sprouts and individual sprouts anastomose with each other to form capillary loops, which then elongate and may be the source of additional sprouts. It is clear that angiogenesis is entirely the result of endothelial cell proteolytic, migratory and proliferative activity.

Tumour Angiogenesis: The Pathologist's Point of View

Malignant tumours grow rapidly and thus have a greater need of oxygen and nutrients than do normal tissues. This need is met by a rich supply of newly formed tumour vessels. Virchow, as long ago as 1863, commented on the abnormal number of capillaries in malignant neoplasms [22]. The importance of vascularisation for tumour growth was shown by Folkman and his colleagues, who transplanted neoplasms into isolated perfused organs and showed that such transplants not only failed to vascularize, but also stopped growing when they had attained a diameter of 2–3 mm [8, 9]. The failure of vascularisation of the tumour implant appeared to be a consequence of the endothelial cell degeneration in the host tissues, a feature commonly seen in isolated perfused organs. Despite the cessation of growth of the non-vascularized neoplastic implants, their reimplantation back into donor mice resulted in their vascularization and rapid growth. The concept thus arose, and is now firmly established, that there are two phases in tumour development: an initial avascular phase which permits growth only up to a diameter of about 2 mm and a subsequent vascular phase which allows for unlimited growth.

The first indication that this marked vascularity of tumours was due to the secretion of an angiogenic factor by the neoplasm itself came from studies of isolated tumour implants in millipore chambers in the hamster cheek pouch; these showed that the neoplasm was capable of inducing new vascular growth on the opposite side of the filter, a finding suggesting tumour secretion of an angiogenic factor. Further studies utilised the rabbit cornea or the chick chorioallantoic membrane to study tumour-induced angiogenesis, and it was shown that angiogenic activity is acquired, or markedly increased, during the progression of normal cells to the neoplastic state [8].

Tumour-Derived Angiogenic Factors

There have been numerous proposed candidates for the role of tumour-derived angiogenic factor [10], but most have failed to meet the requirement of being both diffusable and having a direct effect on endothelial cells. Several of the candidate substances, which include epidermal growth factor, transforming growth factors alpha and beta, tumour necrosis factor, angiogenin and prostaglandin E_2, are angiogenic in vivo but have no direct mitogenic effect on endothelial cells, and their action is thought to be mediated by other inducers. Basic and acidic fibroblastic growth factors induce endothelial cell proliferation, but lack a hydrophobic signal peptide required for extracellular transport and therefore cannot be the diffusible factor required for tumour angiogenesis; the same point argues against platelet-derived endothelial cell growth factor being the neoplastic angiogenic agent.

Within recent years a secreted disulphide-linked dimeric glycoprotein known as vascular permeability factor, or vascular endothelial growth factor, has been identified in the conditioned media of rodent and human tumour cell lines [6, 14, 17, 20]. This diffusable glycoprotein, which has a limited but distinct homology with platelet-derived growth factor, binds specifically to receptors on vascular endothelial cells [21] and is capable of inducing endothelial cell migration, endothelial cell proliferation and neoangiogenesis [23]. The gene for this substance is not confined to neoplastic cells, but is also found in cells of many normal tissues, such as lung, kidney, heart and adrenal gland [3]. Nevertheless, particularly high levels of expression of this gene have been detected in several human tumours [19], and currently this glycoprotein is the most probable candidate for the role of principal tumour angiogenic factor.

Characteristics of Tumour Vasculature

Tumour blood vessels differ morphologically from normal vessels insofar as they often pursue a tortuous pathway, are not infrequently saccular, are distributed heterogenously throughout the neoplasm and lack contractile wall elements [12]. Furthermore, tumour blood vessels show an altered reactivity to vasoactive agents, having a decreased sensitivity to endothelin, platelet activating factor and angiotensin II [1]. They are particularly unresponsive to vasodilator agents, suggesting that the tumour vascular bed is in a state of near-maximal vasodilatation [18].

Control of Tumour Blood Flow

Maintenance of blood flow is clearly an important factor in sustaining tumour growth. This is achieved, as noted above, at an optimal level by sustained vasodilatation, and it has been suggested that the agent responsible for this is the naturally occurring vasodilator agent nitric oxide. Immunoreactivity for nitric oxide synthase of inducible type is detectable in the endothelial cells of tumour implants in mice after, but not before, the seventh day of implantation, but is not found in non-neoplastic implants, in areas of tissue around the implants or in the neoplastic cells [4]. This finding has been complemented by functional studies which have shown that local inhibition of nitric oxide production in a murine tumour implant, by substances such as methylene blue or arginine analogues, results in a marked reduction of tumour blood flow [2]. It thus appears that tumours can maintain their blood flow by inducing the generation of nitric oxide synthase in the endothelium of their blood vessels. The mechanism by which this is achieved is, however, currently obscure.

Vascular Patterns in Gynaecological Neoplasms

It has to be admitted that no corpus of information regarding the degree of vascularity or the pattern of vascularization of gynaecological neoplasms exists in the pathological literature. There have been no systematic surveys of tumour vascularity, no morphometric analyses of tumour blood vessel content and few, if any, microinjection studies of neoplasms of the female genital tract. This apparent indifference of pathologists to tumour vascularization reflects the extremely limited diagnostic importance of blood vessels in tumour histopathology. It is, of course, well recognized that most malignant neoplasms have a well-marked, and atypical, vessel content and that the majority of benign neoplasms have a much less striking degree of vascularity, but this difference in vascularization is rarely used by the histopathologist as a diagnostic criterion. There are a few neoplasms which, very characteristically, have a rich vascular content as one of their diagnostic features, these including endometrial stromal sarcomas, ovarian sclerosing stromal tumours, aggressive angiomyxomas of the pelvic soft tissues and the nosologically debatable uterine haemangiopericytomas. Whilst some extremely rare vascular neoplasms, such as angiosarcomas, are diagnosed largely on the basis of their vascular pattern, these are exceptions rather than the rule and it has to be borne in mind that marked vascularity is not an absolute indicator of malignancy, for the highly vascular sclerosing stromal tumours of the ovary are benign whilst many banal leiomyomas of the uterine body have a high content of vessels. Furthermore non-neoplastic lesions, such as inflammatory granulation tissue, endometriosis and ovarian luteal cysts, may contain many vessels.

Despite these many caveats it probably remains true that a rich content of abnormal vessels within a pelvic or adnexal mass is clearly indicative of a malignant lesion and it is, of course, this characteristic of malignant neoplasms which has been most studied by transvaginal colour flow Doppler. It has to be remembered, however, that the vascular pattern of a malignant tumour may be altered by necrosis (which in some malignant neoplasms can be very extensive), by tumour compression of the contained vessels, by tumour cell plugging of vessels and, particularly in the case of ovarian neoplasms, by torsion of the organ.

This paucity of information derived from pathological studies is currently being repaired by transvaginal colour Doppler studies, which are providing new information about gynaecological tumour vascularity (see chapter by Bourne et al. on "The Study of Ovarian Tumours") [5, 7, 11, 13, 15, 24] and which should be stimulating pathologists to study more carefully and more intensively the vasculature of neoplasms which have been removed after Doppler study. It is particularly important that the relatively few malignant tumours which do not show an increased vascularity are subjected to careful histological examination so that an adequate explanation of these "false negatives" is obtained.

Quite apart from the assessment of the degree of vascularity, pathologists also need to undertake topographic analyses of tumour vessels. Doppler studies are identifying central, peripheral, septal, pericystic and intrapapillary areas of vascularization [7, 16], and there is a necessity for histopathological confirmation of the significance of these various vascular patterns.

References

1. Andrade SP, Bakhle YS, Piper PJ (1991) Decreased response to platelet activating factor (PAF), endothelin-1 (ET-1) and angiotensin II (AII) in tumour blood vessels in mice. Br J Pharmacol 104: 422
2. Andrade SP, Hart IR, Piper PJ (1992) Inhibitors of nitric oxide synthase selectively reduce flow in tumour associated neovasculature. Br J Pharmacol 107: 1092–1095

3. Berse B, Brown LF, Van de Water L, Dvorak HF, Senger DR (1992) Vascular permeability factor (vascular endothelial growth factor) gene is expressed differentially in normal tissues, macrophages and tumors. Mol Biol Cell 3: 211–220
4. Buttery LDK, Springall DR, Andrade SP, Riveros-Morenos V, Hart I, Piper DJ, Polak JM (1993) Induction of nitric oxide synthase in the neo-vasculature of experimental tumours in mice. J Pathol 171: 311–319
5. Carter JR, Fowler JM, Carlson JW, Carson LF, Adcock LL, Twiggs LB (1993) Prediction of malignancy using transvaginal color flow Doppler in patients with gynecologic tumors. Int J Gynecol Cancer 3: 279–284
6. Connolly DT, Olander JV, Heuvelman D, Nelson R, Monsell R, Siegel N, Haymore BL, Leimgruber R, Feder J (1989) Human vascular permeability factor: isolation from U937 cells. J Biol Chem 264: 20017–20024
7. Fleisher AC, Rodgers WH, Bhaskava KR, Kepple DM, Worrell JA, Williams L, Jones HW (1991) Assessment of ovarian tumor vascularity with transvaginal color Doppler sonography. J Ultrasound Med 10: 563–568
8. Folkman J (1985) Tumor angiogenesis. Adv Cancer Res 43: 175–203
9. Folkman J, Cotran R (1976) Relation of vascular proliferation to tumor growth. Int Rev Exp Pathol 16: 207–248
10. Folkman J, Klagsburn M (1987) Angiogenic factors. Science 235: 442–447
11. Hamper UM, Sheth S, Abas FM, Rosenhein NB, Aronson D, Kurman RJ (1993) Transvaginal color Doppler sonography of adnexal masses: differences in blood flow impedance in benign and malignant lesions. Am J Radiol 160: 1225–1228
12. Jain RK (1988) Determinant of tumor blood flow. Cancer Res 48: 2641–2658
13. Kawai M, Kano T, Kikkawa F, Maeda O, Oguchi H, Tomoda Y (1992) Transvaginal Doppler ultrasound with color flow imaging in the diagnosis of ovarian cancer. Obstet Gynecol 79: 163–167
14. Keck PJ, Hauser SD, Krivi G, Sanzo K, Warren T, Feuer J, Connolly DT (1989) Vascular permeability factor, an endothelial cell mitogen related to PDGF. Science 246: 1309–1312
15. Kurjak A, Zalud I, Alfirevic Z (1991) Evaluation of adnexal masses with transvaginal color ultrasound. J Ultrasound Med 10: 295–299
16. Kurjak A, Predanic M, Kupesic-Urek S, Jukic S (1993) Transvaginal color and pulsed Doppler assessment of adnexal tumor vascularity. Gynecol Oncol 50: 3–9
17. Leung DW, Cachianes G, Kuang W-J, Goeddel DV, Ferrara N (1989) Vascular endothelial growth factor is a secreted angiogenic mitogen. Science 246: 1306–1309
18. Peterson HI (1991) Modification of tumour blood flow: a review. Int J Radiat Biol 60: 201–210
19. Plate K, Breier G, Weich H, Risau W (1992) Vascular endothelial growth factor is a potential tumour angiogenesis factor in human gliomas in vivo. Nature 359: 845–848
20. Senger DR, Connolly DT, Peruzzi CA, Alsup D, Nelson R, Leimgruber K, Feder G, Dvorak HF (1987) Purification of vacular permeability factor (VPF) from tumor cell conditioned medium. Fed Proc 46: 2012
21. Vaisman N, Gospodarowicz D, Neufeld G (1990) Characterization of receptors for vascular endothelial growth factor. J Biol Chem 265: 19461–19466
22. Virchow R (1863) Die Krankhaften Geschwulste. Hirschwald, Berlin
23. Wilting J, Christ B, Weich H (1992) The effect of growth factors on the day 134 chorioallantoic membrane (CAM): a study of VEGF (165) and PDGF-BB. Anat Embryol 186: 251–257
24. Weiner Z, Thaler I, Beck D, Rottem S, Deuttchs M, Brandes JM (1992) Diferentiating malignant from benign ovarian tumors with transvaginal color flow imaging. Obstet Gynecol 79: 159–162

Vascular Physiology and Pathophysiology of Early Pregnancy

J. Hustin

Introduction

The period which begins at implantation and ends at the completion of embryonic organogenesis is described as early pregnancy. During these 10–12 weeks the conceptus, i.e. the embryo and its adnexae, is completely buried within the maternal decidua. Contrary to classical theories, it appears that for a substantial period, relations between mother and embryo are limited. There are reasons to believe that a precise equilibrium of local vascular physiology is of paramount importance for the maintenance of a successful pregnancy. Pregnancy is characterized by continuous changes in the volume and weight of the uterus and its contents. Therefore, its blood supply is also modified. It is logical to postulate that local vascular physiology is subject to constant adaptations. These must, however, occur at the right time; failure to do so may lead to pregnancy loss. The first part of this chapter describes the decidual circulation, and the second part, embryonic circulation and some pathophysiological aspects of early human pregnancy.

Uterine Vascular Adaptation to Pregnancy

The spiral arteries within the late secretory endometrium are highly coiled and readily surrounded by a concentric layer of decidual cells (Fig. 1). Soon after implantation, the tortuosity of these arteries increases and they can be traced as a rather dense network around the conceptus.

As soon as the primary trophoblast, i.e. the outer part of the trophoblastic shell comes into contact with the wall of spiral arteries, so-called physiological changes occur. The artery is opened and trophoblastic cells enter it and organize as a loose plug nearly occluding the lumen. Trophoblastic cells drip farther along the vascular lumen in a countercurrent way "like the dripping of wax down the side of a candle" [16].

These trophoblastic plugs are closely linked to the trophoblastic shell and remain so for a considerable period of time. The spiral arteries lose their muscle coat and widen considerably. The new arterial wall is made of cell debris, collagen and other trophoblasts which have moved interstitially and cluster around the vessel.

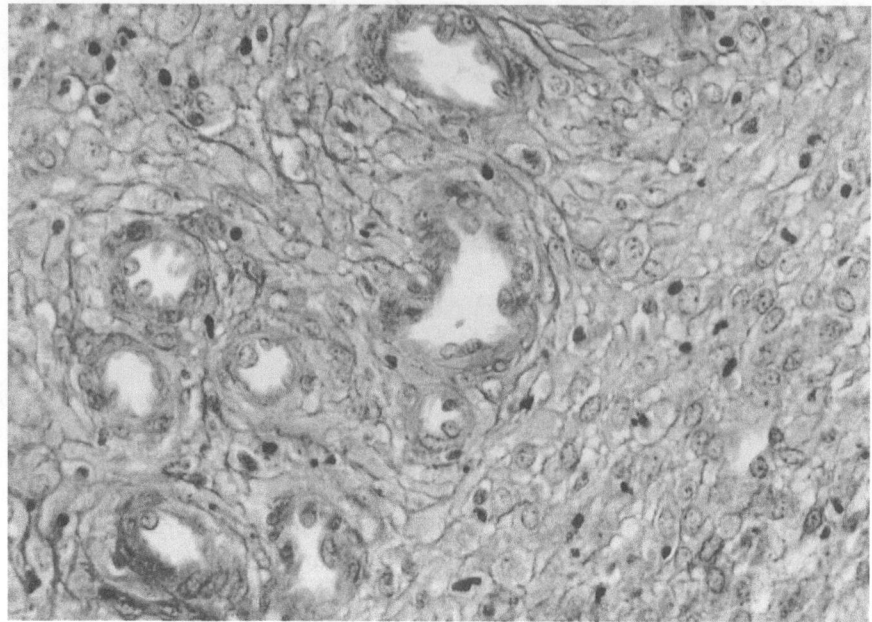

Fig. 1. Spiral artery on day 27 of the cycle. Hematoxylin and eosin, ×400

It is logical to suggest that, during the first few weeks of pregnancy, embryonic requirements are high. However, it seems that free access of maternal blood to the intervillous space is impeded or at least limited [5, 6]. The crucial question is whether there is a true blood flow in the intervillous space during the first 12 weeks and, if not, when it begins.

During the initial steps of interstitial trophoblastic penetration, some endometrial sinusoids are tapped, and for a limited period of time maternal erythrocytes are present in the trophoblastic lacunae. However, ". . . maternal blood in the lacunae, propelled at first only by capillary pressure, moves sluggishly . . ." [16]. We have suggested that the tapped vessels are probably venous sinusoids and that only minute quantities of maternal blood enter the primitive intervillous space in a retrograde fashion [7]. By transvaginal sonography, as well as by perfusion of excised uteri with a pregnancy in situ, we have been unable to demonstrate a free passage of maternal blood in the intervillous space [5, 6, 19]. We believe that the openings of spiral arteries are almost totally occluded by the trophoblastic shell and its outer plugs (Fig. 2). It is highly probable that maternal blood arriving at the deciduo-myometrial junction largely flows via arterio-venous shunts. The remainder percolates between the intravascular trophoblastic cells and is eventually filtered in labyrinthine channels within the trophoblastic shell (Fig. 3). There, leucocytes and red blood cells are efficiently retained, while plasma can escape to the intervillous space. This was readily demonstrated by studies using india ink or barium sulphate uterine perfusion at low pressure [5].

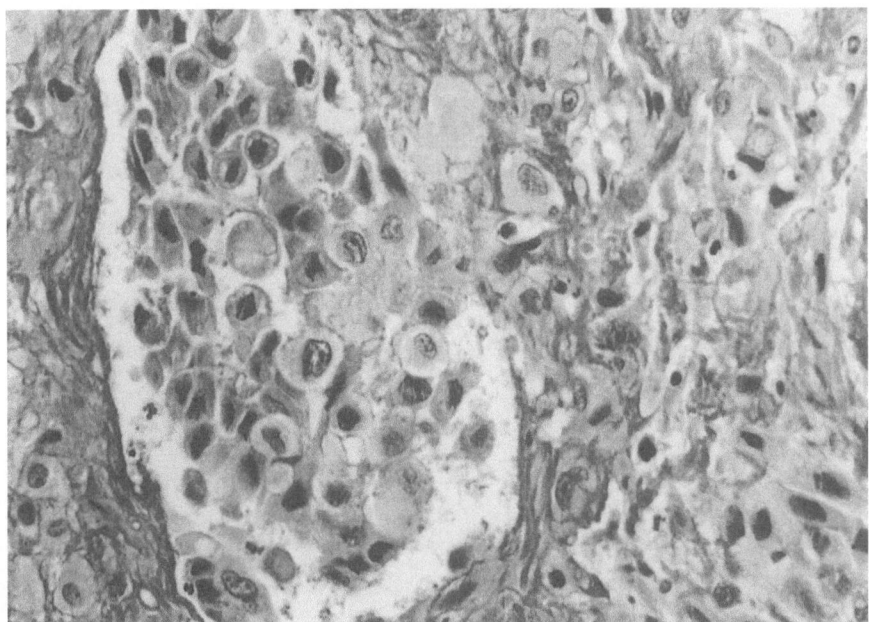

Fig. 2. Utero-placental artery nearly occluded by a trophoblastic plug. Compare the diameter of the vessel with Fig. 1. Hematoxylin and eosin, ×400

Physiologically, it is unlikely that intravascular trophoblastic plugs would not be dislodged if there was significant pressure, and thus a true blood flow, in the utero-placental arteries.

It must be remembered that Boyd and Hamilton [2] have already put forward the hypothesis of a very low blood pressure in the utero-placental arteries and that Moll et al. [12] gave a figure of ±10 mmHg for utero-placental arteries in non-human primates later in gestation. The physiological changes in local arteries and the transformation of the final few millimetres by trophoblast penetration account for such a low figure.

When the decidualization process is completed, the vascular network of the endometrium remote from the implantation area only has a limited importance. During the first trimester, as already mentioned, most of maternal uterine circulation remains within the myometrium, where the flow may be high due to arterio-venous shunts. This phenomenon also explains why during the first 12 weeks so few draining veins are observable at the trophoblastic shell interface.

Embryonic Circulations

It is well established that the first heartbeats occur around day 22 and that the first circulation to be established is embryo-vitelline. [11, 14, 18]. A forward flow is also

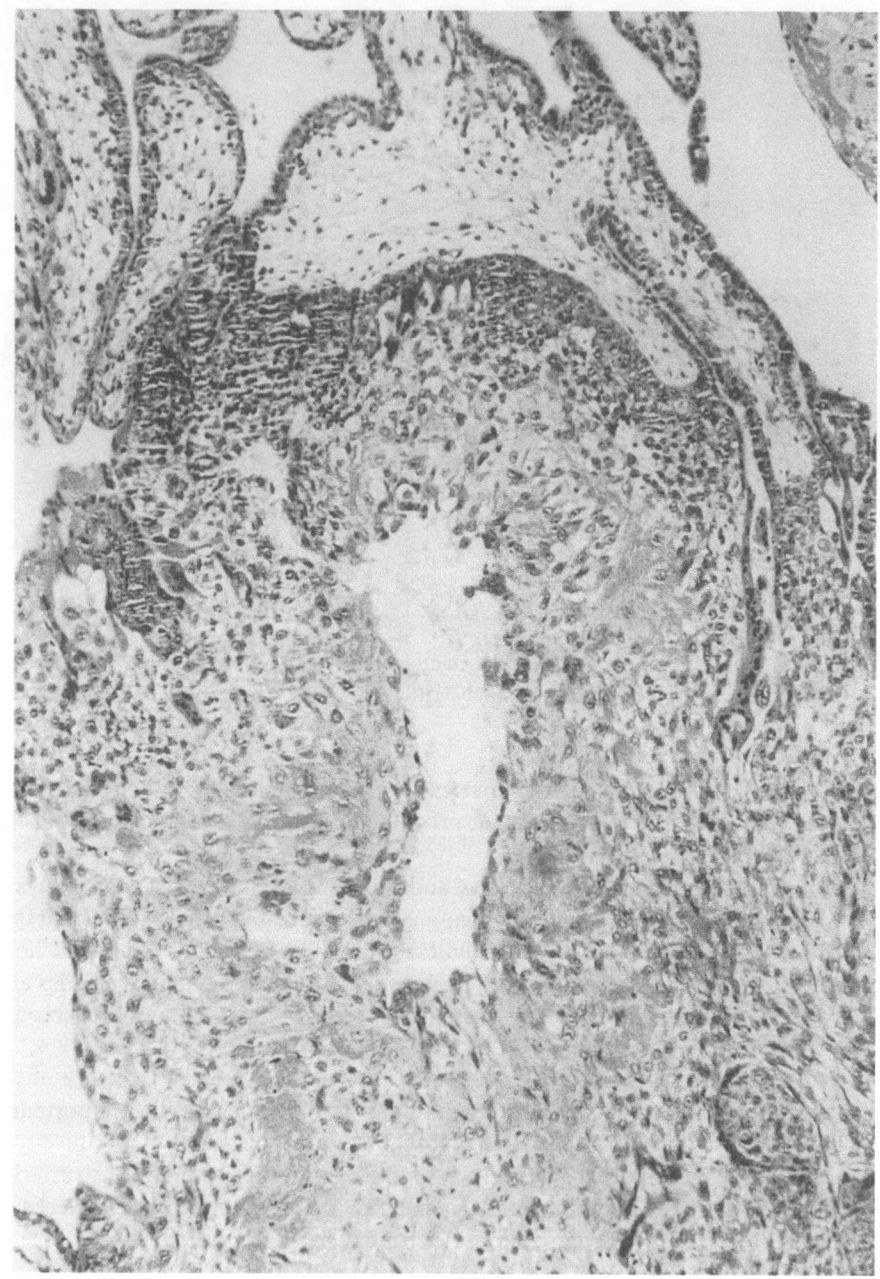

Fig. 3. Materno–embryonic interface. Opening of a utero-placental artery within the labyrinthine channels of the trophoblastic shell. Intervillous space is in the *upper third* of the picture. Hematoxylin eosin, ×63

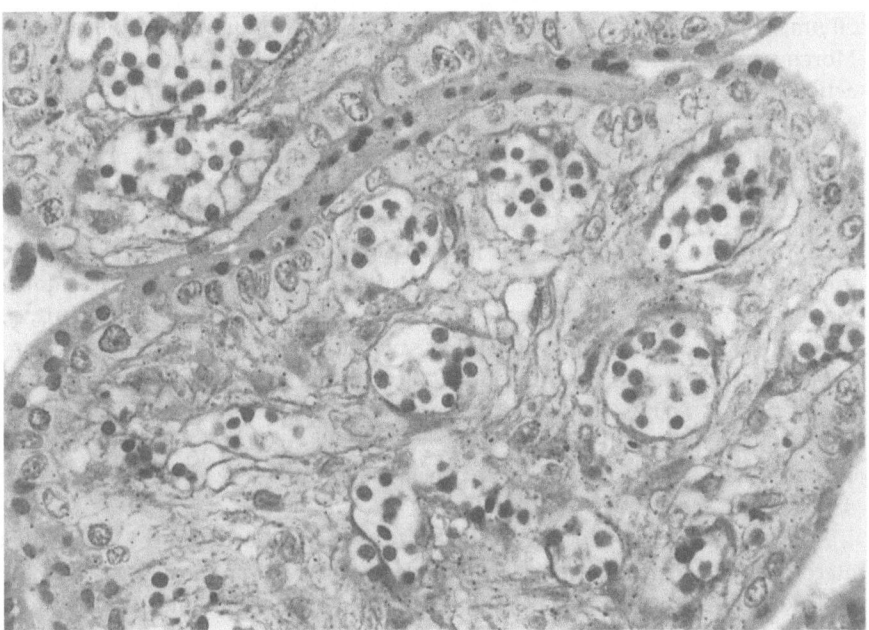

Fig. 4. Early placenta at week 5 of pregnancy. Large villus with capillaries filled with nucleated erythroid cells. Hematoxylin and eosin, ×400

present at this time. It can be postulated that a significant blood volume with a measurable blood pressure (systolic pressure with a stroke volume) is significant around day 24. The yolk-sac communicates with the vascular network of the embryo by two vitelline arteries and veins [8].

Data relative to the cardiovascular physiology of the human embryo are becoming available (see chapter by Wladimiroff and van Splunder, this volume). The diameter of the major vascular trunks is very small; the aorta, for instance, has a maximum diameter of 2 mm at 10 weeks [13].

Experiments on chick embryos, which cannot be extrapolated to human embryos, have shown that systolic pressure varies from 5 mm Hg to 10 mm Hg late in development [18]. However, it is assumed that the blood pressure in human embryos is not higher.

After 4–5 weeks, the circulation incorporates the placental area and villous trees. The yolk-sac is progressively "sequestrated" from the main blood flow and at around 6 weeks the circulation is exclusively embryo-placental (Fig. 4). Obviously, blood pressure within the embryonic circulation must be quite low, as blood volume is also minimal.

However, the embryo must compete with pressures from outside in order to provide a complete flow within the villous capillaries; there, the intravascular tone must be at least equal to the interstitial villous pressure plus the intervillous space pressure. The intervillous space is a very small cavity during the first trimester, and in ideally fixed specimens the distance between contiguous villi does not exceed

20 μm; therefore, it can be suggested that filling with fluid cannot be complete. Moreover, this filling action must occur very slowly due to the extensive filter action of the trophoblastic shell. This can only be achieved if no free blood flow exists.

During the first few weeks of pregnancy, the amniotic cavity is much smaller than the extra-embryonic coelom. Both cavities are filled with fluid, but not to the extent of ballooning the conceptus. The intra-amniotic pressure has been shown to be equal to the intravillous pressure later in pregnancy [4], probably after 12 weeks, when the amniotic cavity expands tremendously. Therefore, it follows that the equilibrium within the whole conceptus, i.e. the embryo and its adnexae, requires external forces, i.e. the uterine inter-stitial pressure plus that within utero-placental arteries to be near zero value or efficiently counterbalanced by embryonic ones. To achieve this goal, the whole conceptus, completely covered by the trophoblastic shell, is only partially inflated and could absorb any pressure changes by simple deformation.

In 1960, Assali et al. declared that "it is generally believed that the fetus in utero lives in a hypoxic state" [1]. They also suggested that the adjustment of the fetus to the low oxygen tension could be achieved by a tremendously high systemic blood flow, a very high oxygen extraction by fetal tissues, a particularly elevated oxygen capacity of fetal blood and probably also by a distinct property of the fetus to adjust to an anaerobic metabolism.

Primitive haematopoiesis begins in the yolk-sac either during the fifth week of gestation [8] or even earlier [20]. Within the extra-embryonic cell islands, progenitor cells differentiate as nucleated erythroid cells (erythroblasts) [22]. These nucleated cells are loaded with embryonic haemoglobins, i.e. Hb Gower I and II (with zeta-2) epsilon-2 and alpha-2 epsilon-2 chains, respectively) and minute amounts of Hb Portland (zeta-2 gamma-2) [15, 21]. These embryonic haemoglobins have been shown to have a very high affinity for oxygen at the low concentrations of interstitial fluids [9, 23]. In addition, the metabolism of early embryos is clearly not the same as in more developed fetuses or adults. In fact, Wells et al. [23] have shown that the embryonic energy requirement is significantly lower in early mouse embryos. Recently, Rodesch et al. [17] demonstrated that in normal first-trimester human preg-nancies, placental pO_2 remained significantly lower than the endometrial levels, although this difference almost disappeared after 12 weeks. Another important fact is that, in vitro, early embryos will develop significantly better under reduced pO_2 [10].

It is thus quite possible that the hypothesis of Assali et al. [1] of a predominently anaerobic metabolism of the embryo reflects the truth. Conceiv-ably, a highly efficient embryo-placental circulation is needed to provide the basic requirements. There are obvious similarities between cardiovascular and meta-bolic adjustments of the early embryo and the physiology of oxygen transfer in fish (and their embryos), which can rely solely on the minute amounts of gas dissolved in water [3, 7].

Physiopathological Considerations

The establishment of a successful pregnancy is linked to a state of equilibrium between the conceptus, i.e. placental and embryonic growth, on one hand and uterine distensibility and lowering of interstitial pressures on the other hand. The etiologies of pregnancy loss during the first trimester are manifold. However, the mechanisms involved in the process of spontaneous abortion most probably derive from circulatory disturbances either on the maternal side, the embryonic side or both.

It is conceivable that the vascular tone of maternal spiral arteries increases and that the intravascular pressure is therefore abnormally elevated. According to our hypothesis, trophoblast plugs are easily dislodged and maternal blood can pour out of the vessel, repelling the trophoblast shell and creating a haemorrhagic cleavage line within the decidua. A similar pathogenic mechanism can be proposed if for any reason arterio-venous shunts at the deciduo-myometrial junction are not open and do not divert the blood flow.

Many cases of spontaneous abortion present as genetic abnormalities. One important feature in these cases is trophoblastic hypoplasia, i.e. the villous cytotrophoblastic layer is considerably reduced in thickness. The trophoblastic shell is also considerably thinned and discontinuous with a markedly diminished number of intravascular trophoblastic plugs [5]. Therefore, a significant blood flow exists within spiral arteries. This also leads to a similar sequence of events and eventually to haemorrhagic dislodging of the conceptus. If the spiral arteries do not undergo all the physiological changes, perhaps because of a deficient trophoblastic invasion, a relatively elevated vascular tone is maintained and the pathogeny of abortion may associate embryonic and maternal factors. In such cases, histological evidence also frequently points to an untimely blood flow in the intervillous space.

Clots are often conspicuous together with necrosis of adjacent villi. Embryonic death follows the considerable increase in intervillous space pressure. Two mechanisms are probably involved: either there is abruptio due to haemorrhagic necrosis of the decidua or there is extravasation of blood within the intervillous space, probably due to tearing of the trophoblastic shell.

Another hypothesis suggests that even when a normal conceptus eventually develops with a normal embryo and an efficient placenta, embryonic death may still occur. In such cases, one has to postulate that a prolonged impairment in the embryo-placental circulation has occurred, probably at the villous capillary level. One explanation is that for one reason or another the pressure in the intervillous space increases and becomes higher than the villous capillary pressure. This leads to immediate closure of the villous capillary bed and to arrest of the embryo-placental circulation, i.e. to embryonic death. It is logical to postulate that in such cases the placenta may survive for a significant period without any significant changes, notably at the deciduo-trophoblastic interface.

We have already postulated [5] that different etiologies could be attributed to the main pathogenic mechanisms of pregnancy loss. These are summarized in Fig.

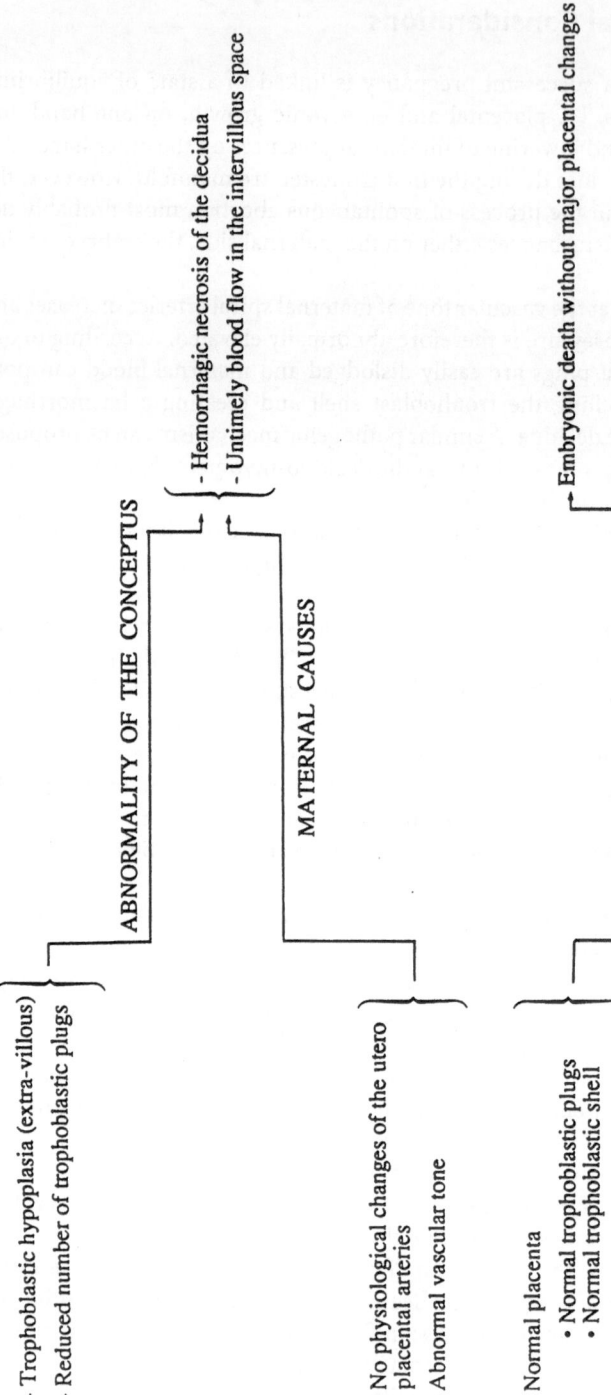

Fig. 5. Possible mechanisms of spontaneous abortion

5. The etiology of spontaneous abortion may remain undetermined in a number of cases. However, histological examination of the conceptus is still extremely useful; it seems to us that determining whether the cause is maternal, embryonic or both may point either to failure or insufficiency of placentation or to an insufficiency of gestational changes within the uterus. Such a diagnosis could in turn lead to more precise etiological investigations and possibly to treatment proposals.

References

1. Assali N, Rauramo L, Peltonen T (1960) Measurement of uterine blood flow and uterine metabolism. VIII. Uterine and fetal blood flow and oxygen consumption in early human pregnancy. Am J Obstet Gynecol 79: 86–98
2. Boyd JD, Hamilton WJ (1970) The human placenta. Heffer, Cambridge
3. Exalto N, Te Velde J, Sarstadt T (1993) The human yolk-sac. Orgyn 4: 9–11
4. Hendricks CH, Quilligan EJ, Tyler CW, Tucker GJ (1959) Pressure relationships between the intervillous space and the amniotic fluid in human term pregnancy. Am J Obstet Gynecol 77: 1028–1037
5. Hustin J, Jauniaux E (1992) Morphology and mechanisms of abortion. In: Barnea ER, Hustin J, Jauniaux E (eds) The first twelve weeks of gestation. Springer, Berlin Heidelberg New York, pp 280–296
6. Hustin J, Schaaps JP, Lambotte R (1988) Anatomical studies of the utero-placental vascularization in the first trimester of pregnancy. Trophoblast Res 3: 49–60
7. Hustin J (1992) The materno-trophoblastic inferface: uteroplacental blood flow. In: Barnea ER, Hustin J, Jauniaux E (eds) The first twelve weeks of gestation. Springer, Berlin Heidelberg New York, 97–110
8. Jauniaux E, Moscoso JG (1992) Morphology and significance of the human yolk-sac. In: The first twelve weeks of gestation. Barnea ER, Hustin J, Jauniaux E (eds) Springer, Berlin Heidelberg New York, pp 192–213
9. Kaplan LA, Pesce AJ (1984) Clinical chemistry: theory, analysis and correlation. Mosby, St Louis, pp 623–624
10. Khurana NK, Wales RG (1989) Effect of oxygen concentration on the metabolism of [u-^{14}C] glucose by mouse morulae and early blastocysts in vitro. Reprod Fertil Dev 1: 99–106
11. Larsen WJ (1993) Human embryology. Churchill Livingstone, New York
12. Moll W, Künzel, Herberger J (1975) Hemodynamic implications of hemochorial placentation. Eur J Obstet Reprod Biol 5: 67–74
13. Moscoso JG (1992) Functional aspects of Embryology. In: Barnea ER, Hustin J, Jauniaux E (eds) The first twelve weeks of gestation. Springer, Berlin Heidelberg New York, pp 169–191
14. O'Rahilly R, Müller F (1992) Human embryology and teratology. Wiley/Liss, New York
15. Peschle C, Mavilio F, Care A, Migliaccio G, Migliaccio AR, Salvo G, Samoggia P, Petti S, Guerriero R, Marinucci M, Lazzaro D, Russo G, Mastroberardino G (1985) Haemoglobin switching in human embryos: asynchrony of $\zeta \to \alpha$ and $\varepsilon \to \gamma$-globin switches in primitive and definitive erythropoietic lineage. Nature 313: 235–237
16. Ramsey E, Donner MW (1988) Placental vasculature and circulation in primates. Trophoblast Res 3: 217–233
17. Rodesch F, Simon PH, Donner C, Jauniaux E (1992) Oxygen measurements in endometrial and trophoblastic tissues during early pregnancy. Obstet Gynecol 80: 283–285
18. Ruckman RN, O'Brien SA, Messersmith DJ (1988) Functional development of the heart: hemodynamics. In: Meisami E, Timiras PS (eds) Handbook of human growth and developmental biology, vol IIIB. CRC Press, Boca Raton, pp 69–84

19. Schaaps JP, Hustin J (1988) In vivo aspects of the materno-trophoblastic border during the first trimester of gestation. Trophoblast Res 3: 39–48
20. Schnall SF, Benz EJ (1990) Developmental patterns of human hemoglobin synthesis. In: Meisami E, Timiras PS (eds) Handbook of human growth and developmental biology, vol IIIA. CRC Press, Boca Raton, pp 135–147
21. Shahidi NT, Ershler WB (1990) Developmental changes in blood as a whole. In: Meisami E, Timiras PS (eds) Handbook of human growth and developmental biology, vol IIIA. CRC Press, Boca Raton, pp 77–100
22. Tavassoli M (1990) Ontogeny of hemopoiesis. In: Meisami E, Timiras PS (eds) Handbook of human growth and developmental biology, vol III A. CRC Press, Boca Raton, pp 101–112
23. Wells RM, Trevenen BJ, Brittain T (1989) Adenylate energy charge and hemoglobin function in developing mouse embryos. Comp Biochem Physiol [B] 92(2): 365–367

New Diagnostic and Therapeutic Approaches to Gestational Trophoblastic Tumours

J.E. Boultbee and E.S. Newlands

Introduction

Gestational trophoblastic tumours (GTT) are unique in cancer biology since genetically they are either partially or completely paternally derived. GTT may occur after any form of pregnancy, but the most common presentation is with a hydatidiform mole (HM). The classical hydatidiform mole (CHM) is an androgenetic conceptus where the maternal genes have been deleted and the abnormal pregnancy presents between 8 and 12 weeks into gestation with vaginal bleeding and florid hydropic villi of trophoblast in the uterus and myometrium. Partial hydatidiform mole (PHM) is a triploid conceptus and again presents with vaginal bleeding, but with much less florid hydropic change in the trophoblastic villi; it commonly has some evidence of foetal development pathologically. Choriocarcinoma is a frank malignancy of the trophoblast and is an extremely vascular tumour, rapidly metastasising through the venous system to the lungs, brain and other sites. The incidence of malignancy following CHM is approximately 8% in the Charing Cross series and 0.5% after PHM. Choriocarcinoma can occur after molar pregnancies, full-term pregnancies and abortions. Over the last decade, a rare variant of choriocarcinoma, placental site trophoblastic tumour (PSTT), has been recognised pathologically and clinically. This tends to be a less widely metastasising tumour than choriocarcinoma and infiltrates locally in the pelvis.

In the United Kingdom, patients at risk of developing a GTT are registered with the national screening service and registered at three reference laboratories in Dundee, Sheffield and the Charing Cross Hospital in London. Approximately 1200 women are registered annually, and of these approximately 100 will need chemotherapy because their post-molar trophoblastic disease has not died out or is causing complications of vaginal haemorrhage. The prognosis for these patients is now excellent with appropriate management and it has been important to integrate new diagnostic techniques into the staging and management of these patients. The treatment of patients with GTT is mainly by chemotherapy and, in selected cases, surgery if there is evidence of drug resistance.

Prognostic Factors for Therapy

Patients are selected for treatment on the basis of a range of prognostic factors which have been recognised over the last 30 years. The major adverse prognostic factors recognised in these patients are:

1. High-level marker hormone of this group of diseases, human chorionic gonadotrophin (hCG), in the serum and urine (more than 100 000 IU/l in serum).
2. The duration the disease has been present in the patient. If the disease has been persisting for more than 12 months, there is a tendency for the tumour to become drug resistant.
3. Widely metastatic disease (pulmonary, brain, liver and other sites).
4. Failure of prior chemotherapy significantly increases the risk of developing drug resistance.

At the Charing Cross Hospital we categorise patients into low, medium and high risk in terms of the chance of their tumour developing drug resistance. Patients with low-risk disease are treated with methotrexate and folinic acid, which is simple, non-toxic and does not induce alopecia. The medium-risk patients need a sequence of drugs to eliminate their disease, and high-risk patients are treated with drug combinations from the outset [7, 8]. The largest group of patients, those falling into the low-risk category, need to be monitored carefully through their treatment, since one in four will need to change from methotrexate to more intensive chemotherapy because of the development of drug resistance [9].

Use of Grey-Scale Imaging

We have routinely used ultrasound for 15 years in all new patients treated for GTT at Charing Cross. As ultrasound has developed in sophistication, this has given increasingly accurate delineation of the uterine size, vascularity and pelvic extent of disease. The two-dimensional ultrasound appearances of GTT tumours are non-specific, and similar appearances may be seen in HM, hydropic degeneration, degenerating fibroids and ovarian dysgerminomas [16]. The uterine size can vary considerably; we have seen uterine volumes as high as 600 cc in large tumours and very small tumours in uteri below 100 cc in volume. Most of these lesions within the uterus or parametria are focal; however, diffuse spread may be present, especially in the vaginal wall. It must also be remembered that an abnormally high uterine volume may be present with a co-existing uterine fibroid. The differention between GTT and a fibroid is difficult, since their grey-scale appearances are very similar and even on colour Doppler areas of increased vascularity may sometimes cause confusion [12]. Ultrasound is also useful in detecting hepatic metastases, which have an adverse prognosis. We analysed 153 low-risk patients with GTT between 1988 and 1990. Ultrasound estimation of the pelvis is available for 88% of these patients and the uterine pulsatility index (PI) for 56% of these. A total of 77

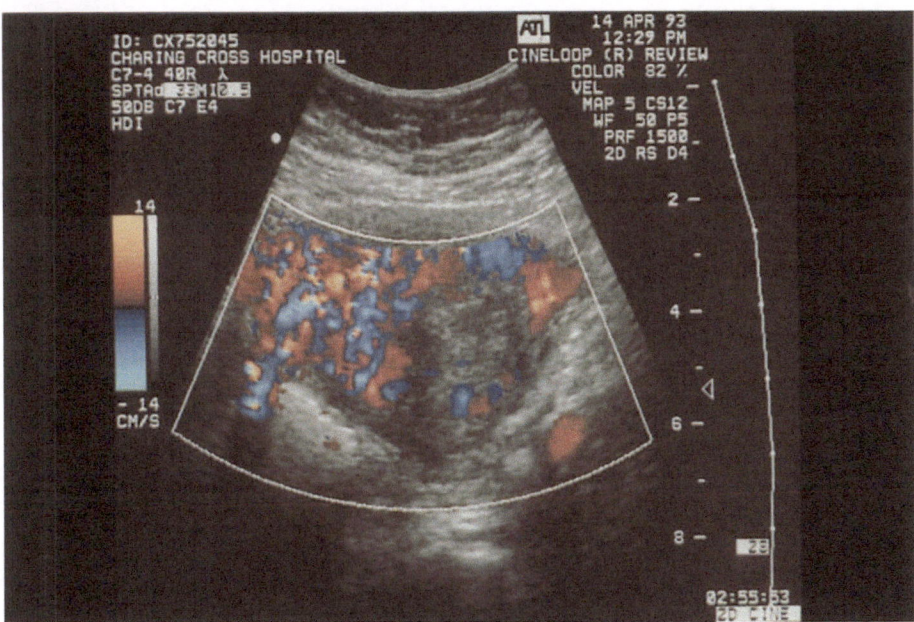

Fig. 1. Transverse colour Doppler (CD) scan of the uterus in a patient with gestational trophoblastic tumour (GTT). The flow from the right uterine artery is increased and there is a typical vascular pattern produced by arterio-venous shunting

patients had an enlarged uterus (larger than 120 ml) on their pre-treatment scan. In this series the PI did not predict the development of drug resistance. However, in a multivariate analysis the two features that were detected as predictors of the development of drug resistance to methotrexate were an enlarged uterus (a volume greater than 120 ml) and a serum hCG of more than 10^4 IU/l. So far this recent information has not been integrated into our prognostic system, but probably should be in the near future. The contribution of ultrasound in assessing the disease in the pelvis is clearly much more useful than clinical examination, which is unable to assess the full extent of the disease. GTT are highly vascular and ideally suited to imaging with colour Doppler, which displays the abnormal blood vessels and their circulation (Figs. 1, 2) [14]. Many of the larger tumours appear as arterio-venous fistulae, and for this transabdominal colour Doppler scanning is often sufficient without transvaginal scanning because of the large area of tissue to be examined and the high velocities being sampled (Fig. 3).

Use of Doppler

The character of the increase in blood flow has been well recognised in ultrasound studies of these conditions, as they create high-velocity, low-resistance vascular beds similar to those seen in pregnancy [5]. The enlarged spiral arteries enter

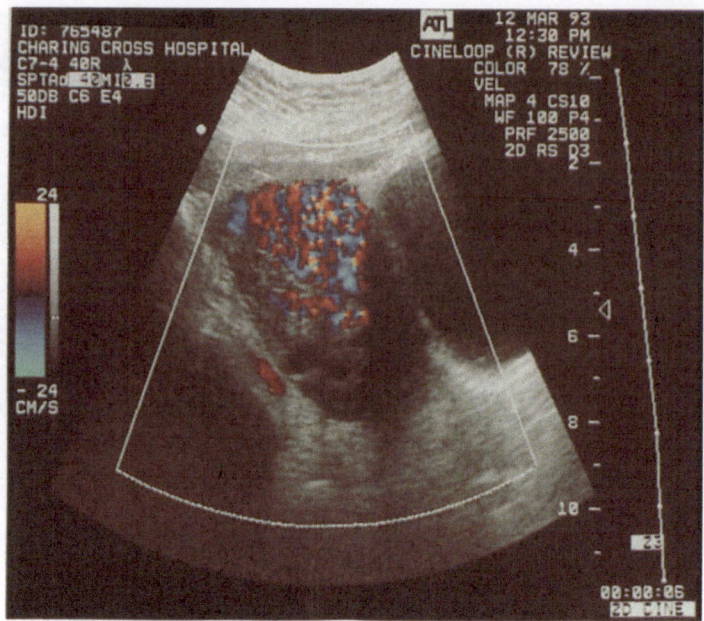

Fig. 2. Longitudinal colour Doppler (CD) scan of the uterus showing a significant fundal and uterine tumour

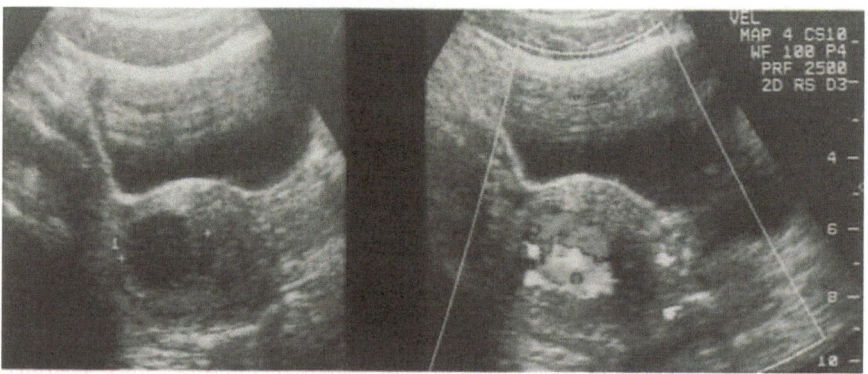

Fig. 3. Two transverse scans of the same uterus with a 3-cm tumour. The *left* scan without colour Doppler (CD) shows an echo-free, well-defined focal area. The *right* scan with CD switched on demonstrates a characteristic flow pattern filling the tumour

venous lakes, allowing early venous return, and the result is an increase in the blood flow, which is expressed as high systolic velocities associated with an increase in diastolic flow, which in turn results in low impedance. Studies of the normal uterine artery in non-pregnant women [7] show a high impedance to flow; PI vary between 1.21 and 5.29. Using transvaginal Doppler [11] and transvaginal colour flow Doppler [15], it has been shown that blood flow impedance within the main uterine artery varies during the ovarian and menstrual cycles [13]. In invasive mole and choriocarcinoma, the PI are significantly lower than in the non-pregnant uterus, although the PI of the uterine arteries in pregnancies at between 10 and 16 weeks can be lower than in GTT [5]. The myometrial signals may not be as diffuse or of such a high intensity as they are in GTT.

Low impedance flow present in the first trimester is seen at the site of placental development, with the main uterine artery still displaying a high impedance flow, as evidenced by a notch in the waveform. In most cases the difference between early pregnancy and abortion on the one hand and GTT on the other should be apparent because of the irregular pattern of flow in the latter. Very small focal tumours have often been difficult to differentiate when the uterine artery demonstrates a high impedance to flow. Colour Doppler has considerably improved the sensitivity of detection of small tumours and the overall scan time in our department. We found that our scan time was decreased by 50% and sensitivity increased when compared with duplex Doppler scanning [10]. In a group of 20 patients who had lesions, two focal lesions identified on colour Doppler which had increased vascularity and a normal grey-scale pattern were missed on duplex scanning [2].

At the initial ultrasound examination, Doppler has been used routinely to assess the blood flow. It has been our routine in patients with abnormal pelvic ultrasounds to repeat this 6 weeks after completing treatment. In the majority of patients with uterine enlargement at the start of treatment, the uterus has decreased in size after completing treatment, although the uterine volume may not have returned to normal if the initial size is very large. After successful treatment with no clinical or biochemical evidence of active residual tumour and no increase risk of recurrence, the appearance of the uterus and the ovaries in the majority of patients have an abnormal pattern. Persistent cysts may be present in the ovaries. The uterine appearance is variable, with relatively non-specific patterns of hypoechogenicity, hyperechogenicity and mixed patterns. None of these patterns have provided a prognostic guide to the likelihood of recurrence following chemotherapy [4]. In the uterus these features were considered to represent necrotic tumour, haemorrhage or blood clot [1].

New Therapeutic Approach

Concurrent with these abnormal grey-scale appearances, the trophoblast of GTT which stimulates abnormal vascularity in the site of initial disease may persist, leaving an area of greatly increased flow in part of the myometrium. In the majority of these cases, this increased uterine flow does not cause vaginal bleeding and surprisingly seems to cause very little trouble in subsequent pregnancies. However, in a small number of cases, persistent heavy uterine bleeding from these abnormal vessels can present major clinical problems. In this context, if the patient does not wish to have any more children, then the treatment of choice is hysterectomy. However, in some of those wanting to have further pregnancies, the bleeding can be controlled by administering a continuous hormonal contraceptive. If bleeding persists despite this, embolisation of the uterine arteries can be sufficiently successful in controlling the blood flow to prevent further heavy bleeding. Normal pregnancies have occurred following this technique. A good example of this is illustrated in Fig. 4; the patient successfully completed treatment and over 1 year later presented with spontaneous profuse vaginal bleeding. Ultrasound examination demonstrated a considerable increase in uterine artery flow with concurrent low impedance signals from the myometrium (Fig. 4). Arteriography confirmed the Doppler findings of an increase in size of the uterine arteries and extensive perfusion of the myometrium (Fig. 5). Post-embolisation films of the uterine vessels (Fig. 5) show a significant reduction in myometrial perfusion. These findings were confirmed by Doppler examination. In the ensuing weeks, this patient was monitored by clinical assessment and follow-up Doppler examination [3].

GTT occasionally present subtle diagnostic problems. Pelvic ultrasound can help in several clinical situations. In some patients the nature and timing of the antecedent pregnancy to a GTT can be quite uncertain when a patient presents with a rising hCG and no evidence of an intra- or extra-uterine pregnancy. If no histology is available on dilatation and curettage and if there is a very vascular area

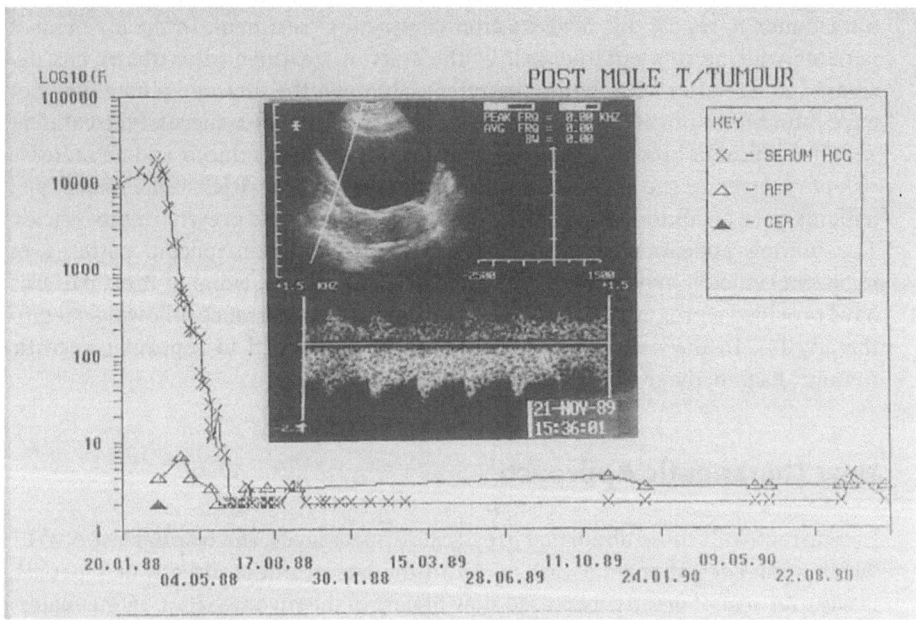

Fig. 4. This patient was treated for post-hydatidiform mole trophoblastic disease in 1988. Although her human chorionic gonadotrophin (hCG) returned to normal, she had heavy vaginal bleeding and required several transfusions in 1989. An ultrasound scan confirmed considerable high-flow characteristics shown on the transverse scan, where the Doppler sample volume is placed on a branch of the right uterine artery

within the uterus, patients sometimes have to be treated with chemotherapy for a presumed GTT in the absence of confirmatory histology. Clearly this policy is only adopted if a hysterectomy is contra-indicated because the patient wants to remain fertile.

Transvaginal colour Doppler is now a well-established technique for assessing the female pelvis. We have found that an increase in the detection rate of GTT has been achieved (Fig. 6). These advantages are best seen when searching for small uterine or extra-uterine masses. The small uterus (less than 150 cc in volume) is easily reviewed and very small tumours, which may be confused with early pregnancy, abortion or ectopic pregnancy, are better shown with the improved grey-scale and colour images.

Some non-gestational tumours can produce hCG, which again presents a diagnostic problem. The clinical pattern of the disease can raise suspicions that the tumour is not gestational in origin, and modern molecular genetic techniques can help if appropriate tissue is available to confirm that the tumour does not contain paternal genes. However, this research technique is not available in most centres, and the absence of an area of increased vascularity in the uterus in these patients as detected by ultrasound and Doppler is one factor in increasing the possibility that the patient has a non-gestational tumour producing hCG. Ectopic pregnancies produce hCG and can present very subtle problems. The combination of ultrasound and Doppler with the pattern of rise in hCG (if this is available) can be very helpful in distinguishing between an ectopic pregnancy and a GTT. While on ultrasound an ectopic pregnancy and a GTT can appear very similar, the rise in HCG is more rapid in an ectopic pregnancy than is usual in the growth of a GTT.

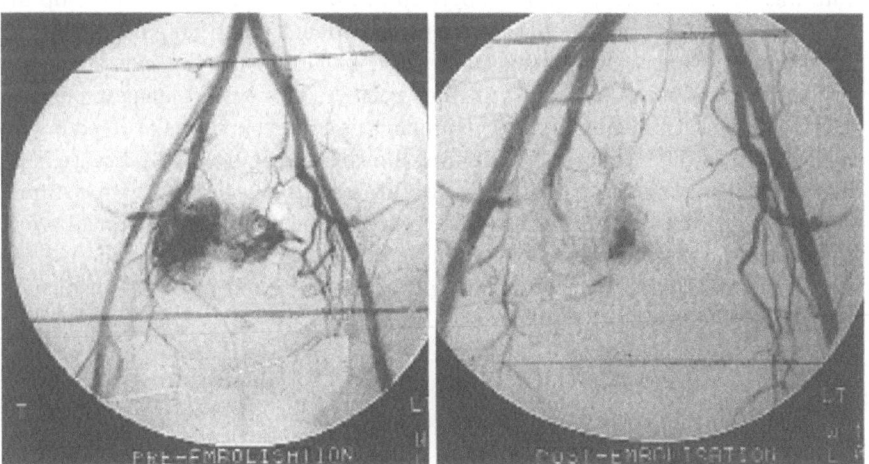

Fig. 5. Pre- and post-embolisation angiograms (*left* and *right*, respectively). After embolisation of the uterine arteries, the patient's bleeding stopped and she had a normal pregnancy in 1991. (Reproduced by kind permission of Dr. J. McIvor)

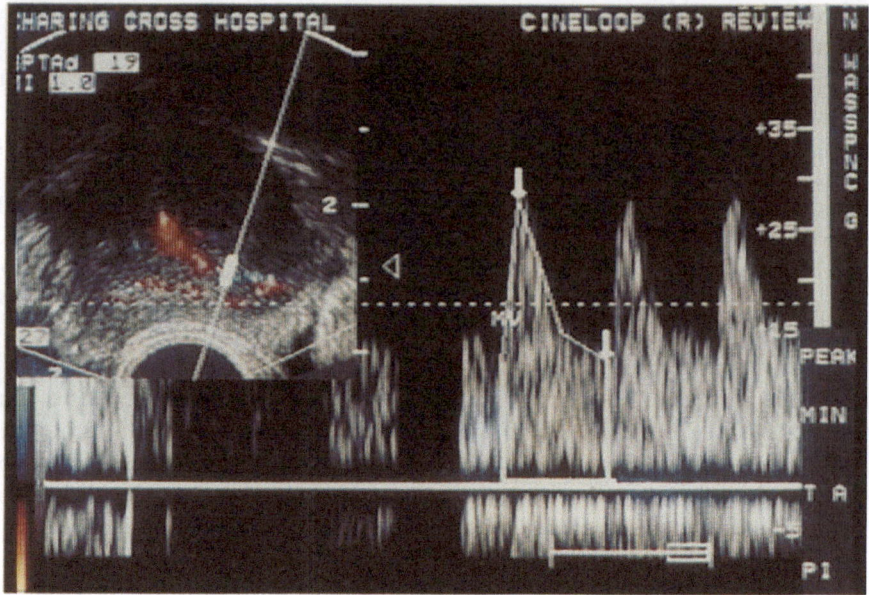

Fig. 6. Colour Doppler (CD) vaginal scan of a very small focal tumour with characteristic increased flow in systole and diastole

Conclusion

The prognosis for patients with GTT is now excellent. In a recent analysis of the Charing Cross series of patients treated since 1979 ($n = 994$), the overall survival rate was 94%. However, a small subgroup of high-risk patients do develop drug resistance and need salvage surgery. In these patients, identifying the site of resistant tumour is important. In this context, pelvic ultrasound can indicate whether or not there is a vascular mass in the uterus, which would suggest persisting uterine disease. Ultrasound is also helpful in this context in terms of detecting liver metastases. In this subgroup of patients, the site of drug-resistant disease is perhaps surprising, since in most cases we are essentially dealing with a tumour starting in the uterus. Although hysterectomy can be useful in individual patients, salvage surgery is clinically more useful in removing drug-resistant disease from the thorax and brain, since in the majority of cases the uterine disease has already been eliminated using chemotherapy.

References

1. Caspi C, Elchalal U, Dgani R, Ben-Hur H, Rozenmam D, Nissim F (1991) Invasive mole and placental site trophoblastic tumor. Ultrasound Med 10: 517–519
2. Dobkin GR, Berkowitz RS, Goldstein DP, Bernstein MR, Doubilet PM (1991) Duplex ultrasonography for persistent gestational trophoblastic tumor. J Reprod Med 36: 14–16

3. Kohorn EI (1993) Evaluation of the criteria used to make the diagnosis of nonmetastatic gestational trophoblastic neoplasia. Gynaecol Oncol 48: 139–147
4. Long MG, Boultbee JE, Begent RHJ, Bagshawe KD (1990) Ultrasonic morphology of the uterus and ovaries after treatment of invasive mole and gestational chorioncarcinoma. Br J Radiol 63: 942–945
5. Long MG, Boultbee JE, Begent RHJ, Hanson ME, Bagshawe KD (1990) Preliminary Doppler studies on the uterine artery and myometrium in trophoblastic tumours requiring chemotherapy. Br J Obstet Gynaecol 97: 686–689
6. Long MG, Boultbee JE, Hanson ME, Begent RHJ (1989) Doppler time velocity waveform studies of the uterine artery and uterus. Br J Obstet Gynaecol 96: 588–593
7. Newlands ES, Bagshawe KD, Begent RHJ (1986) Developments in chemotherapy for medium and high risk patients with gestational trophoblastic tumours (1979–1984). Br J Obstet Gynaecol 93: 63–69
8. Newlands ES, Bagshawe KD, Begent RHJ (1991) Results with the EMA/CO (etoposide, methotrexate, actinomycin D, cyclophosphamide, vincristine) regimen in high risk gestational trophoblastic tumours. 1979 to 1989. Br J Obstet Gynaecol 98: 550–557
9. Newlands ES, Fisher RA, Searle F (1992) The immune system in disease: gestational trophoblastic tumours. In: Stirrat GM, Scott JR (eds) Clinical obstetrics and gynaecology. Bailliere Tindall, London, pp 519–539
10. Rhymer JC, Gwyther SJ, O Reilly SM, Newlands ES, Boultbee JE (1991) Advantages of colour Doppler ultrasound over duplex Doppler ultrasound in the management of gestational trophoblastic tumour. Proceedings of the Royal College of Radiologists
11. Santolaya-Forgas J (1992) Physiology of the menstrual cycle by ultrasonography. Ultrasound Med 11: 139–142
12. Schiller VL, Grant EG (1992) Doppler Ultrasonography of the pelvis. In: Colman G (ed) The radiologic clinics of North America: the female pelvis. Saunders, Philadelphia, pp 735–742
13. Scholtes MCW, Wladimiroff JW, Van Rijen HJM, Hop WCJ (1989) Uterine and ovarian flow velocity wave forms in the normal menstrual cycle: a transvaginal Doppler study. Fertil Steril 52: 981–985
14. Shimamoto K, Sakuma S, Ishigaki T, Makino N (1987) Intratumoral blood flow: evaluation with color Doppler echography. Radiology 165: 683–685
15. Steer CV, Campbell S, Pampiglione JS, Kingsland CR, Mason BA, Collins WP (1990) Transvaginal colour flow imaging of the uterine arteries during the ovarian and menstrual cycles. Hum Reprod 5: 391–395
16. Taylor KJW, Schwartz PE, Kohorn EI (1987) Gestational trophoblastic neoplasia: diagnosis with Doppler US. Radiology 165: 445

II. Uterus

Vascular Changes During the Normal and Artificial Cycle

C.V. STEER

Introduction

In vitro fertilization and embryo transfer (IVF-ET) is a successful infertility treatment with cumulative conception and live birth rates which compare favourably with those of spontaneous conception in the normal fertile population (Fig. 1) [15, 16]. However, despite improvements in fertilization rates and ovarian stimulation regimens, the probability of implantation per embryo transferred has not increased significantly and remains relatively low at between 10% and 15% [3]. Thus the major rate-limiting step in IVF today is a failure of implantation. Clinicians have become like a gardener who spends years developing the best-quality seed (embryos), but takes no care to ensure that the soil (uterus) into which the seed is planted is receptive to provide the correct nutrients for germination (implantation) and growth.

A mathematical model to describe the probability of an embryo implanting has been formulated and contains three variables: embryo transfer efficiency, embryo quality and endometrial receptivity [9]. Paulson et al. concluded that "endometrial receptivity is markedly diminished in ovarian stimulated cycles and is the principle rate limiting step of IVF."

A further statistical model has been developed to study the relative contributions of embryo quality and endometrial receptivity to successful implantation [11]. The mathematically derived values from the analysis of data from four IVF clinics for the contribution of embryo quality ranged from 21% to 32% and for endometrial receptivity from 31% to 64%. Accordingly, a technique that could estimate uterine receptivity might be of value in deciding whether or not cultured embryos should be transferred or whether they should be frozen until the uterus is more receptive. Furthermore, the same information might be used to determine the number of embryos that should be transferred to achieve a singleton pregnancy.

The ultimate test of uterine response in an assisted reproduction cycle would be a non-invasive accurate assessment of physiological normality, preceding the transfer of the embryos. This would allow time to either cryopreserve the embryos or, if this is not acceptable to the patient, to manipulate the hormonal environment in an attempt to achieve an increased probability of conception after embryo transfer. A serum marker of uterine receptivity would be ideal. However, as the embryos are routinely transferred into the uterine cavity 2 days following oocyte

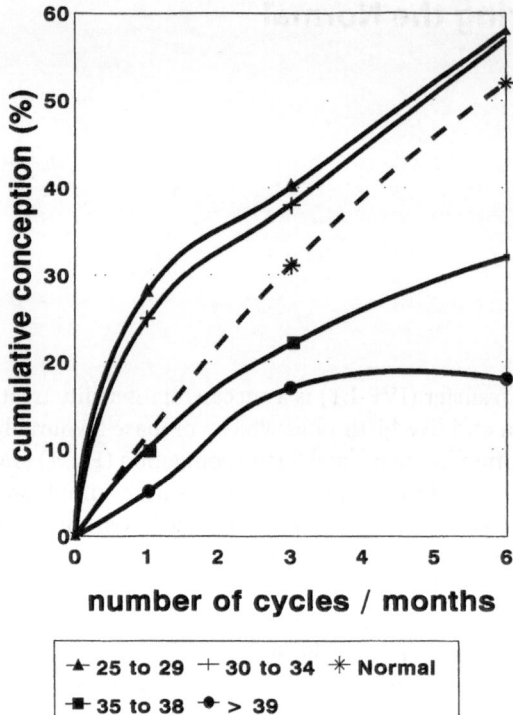

number of cycles / months

Fig. 1. Cumulative conception rate in 4777 in vitro fertilization (IVF) treatment cycles classified by age compared to that of the normal population in the United Kingdom

-▲- 25 to 29   -+- 30 to 34   -*- Normal
-■- 35 to 38   -●- > 39

recovery (ovulation) and implantation occurs around 5 days later, a serum marker of receptivity is unlikely to prove clinically useful.

Methods of Assessing Uterine Receptivity

The search for a suitable indicator of uterine receptivity has ranged from utilizing histological dating criteria from peri-implantation endometrial biopsies [7] to the identification of 63 protein bands by uterine secretion electrophoresis and the pattern of distribution of proteins in the secretory phase of the menstrual cycle [2].

Since the advent of real-time ultrasound, the possibility of monitoring changes in the female reproductive tract by a reproducible, non-invasive, harmless technique has become available. It was first used by the transabdominal transvesical route for demonstrating the growth of ovarian follicles and their subsequent collapse [10], and has subsequently been utilized in assisted reproduction programmes to assess optimal endometrial characteristics pertaining to implantation.

Gonen and colleagues [4] suggested that endometrial thickness on the day before oocyte recovery was significantly greater in the pregnant than the non-pregnant woman and that this may predict the likelihood of implantation. However, other workers have found that measurement of endometrial thickness had no predictive value for pregnancy.

With regard to the endometrial appearance, it has been suggested that a multilayered endometrial pattern (ring) is associated with a significantly higher pregnancy rate [19]. The ultrasound appearance of an endometrial ring is assumed to be due to glandular oedema, and its absence associated with suboptimal uterine conditions for implantation of an embryo. However, the presence of an endometrial ring is a positive or negative phenomenon. Although its presence does suggest a receptive endometrium, it cannot be used as an index to monitor improvement in endometrial conditions.

Uterine Blood Flow

In most of the blood vessels in the body, a high degree of stability is maintained once embryological development is complete. However, the blood vessels to the uterus, and in particular to the endometrium, are highly variable. These variations are of two types: those of the regularly recurring interruptions of the vascular patterns associated with the menstrual cycle, compounded with the upheavals of a pregnancy. The efficiency with which the blood vessels adapt to this changing schedule forms the dividing line between normal physiological function and pathology. The factors that produce vascular variability also control the cyclic changes in the parenchymatous tissues of the endometrium (necessary to enable implantation of an embryo); to a large extent these changes are secondary to those of the blood vessels.

Since the control of uterine blood vessel development also controls the developing endometrium, it is therefore likely that a study of the physiological control of uterine blood supply will produce useful information regarding the optimal conditions required for embryos to implant.

One of the clinically most popular techniques to have been developed for the study of blood flow is Doppler ultrasound velocimetry. An ultrasound beam is used to survey the region of interest, and a signal is detected which is frequency shifted by interaction with the moving blood cells. This method is well established for the study of velocity waveforms in arteries.

The complementary use of transabdominal real-time imaging and pulsed Doppler has demonstrated that characteristic waveforms may be obtained from the uterine arteries of non-pregnant women [17, 18]. The use of transabdominal real-time imaging with an offset Doppler transducer and the calculation of the resistance index suggested that there was increased uterine perfusion during the course of the menstrual cycle, which correlated with rising concentrations of plasma oestradiol and progesterone [6].

The development of endovaginal probes, which involve the use of higher-frequency ultrasound for imaging and pulsed Doppler, have facilitated studies of blood flow in uterine arteries [12].

Transvaginal Colour Doppler of the Normal Cycle

I have shown that endovaginal colour flow imaging can be used to obtain flow velocity waveforms (FVW) from the uterine arteries at any time during the menstrual cycle in apparently healthy women. The use of this technique enables the blood vessels to be easily identified (Fig. 2) and provides an optimal angle for insonation with pulsed Doppler. With the complimentary use of colour Doppler, the ascending branch of the uterine artery can confidently be located just lateral to the cervix. Moreover, the close proximity of the probe to the reproductive organs enables the use of ultrasound at a higher frequency, which produces a greater Doppler shift. These advantages are reflected in a high reproducibility of the pulsatility index, which is an indication of blood flow impedance. Accordingly, it is particularly interesting that the mean times of lowest impedance to uterine blood flow (Fig. 3) occur at the start of rapid follicular growth 6 days before the luteinizing hormone (LH) peak and subsequently during peak luteal function, around the presumed time when implantation might occur. There is also evidence for a short increase in uterine resistance to blood flow around the third day after the LH peak (i.e. around the time of fertilization; Fig. 4). The peak impedance to uterine blood flow around the time of menses (Fig. 5) may be part of the mechanism which regulates the breakdown of the endometrium. Similarly, the increasing impedance to uterine blood flow during the development of a pre-ovulatory follicle may reflect the complex inter-organ regulatory mechanisms which lead to ovulation.

FVW were analyzed in the mid-luteal phase of the menstrual cycle in women with known causes of infertility and were compared with those obtained from women with normal fertility being treated by insemination with donor sperm.

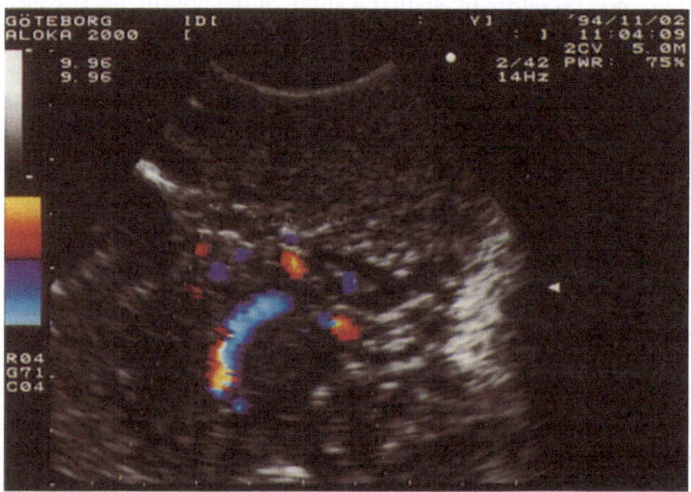

Fig. 2. A longitudinal ultrasound section of the uterus demonstrating the ascending branch of the uterine artery as a pulsating blue colour just lateral to the cervix

When the pulsatility index (PI) values for patients with different causes of infertility were compared with those of the normal women, it was found that patients in all categories of infertility had PI valves that differed significantly from normal PI values. Figure 6 shows the ranges of the mid-luteal PI and the percentage of

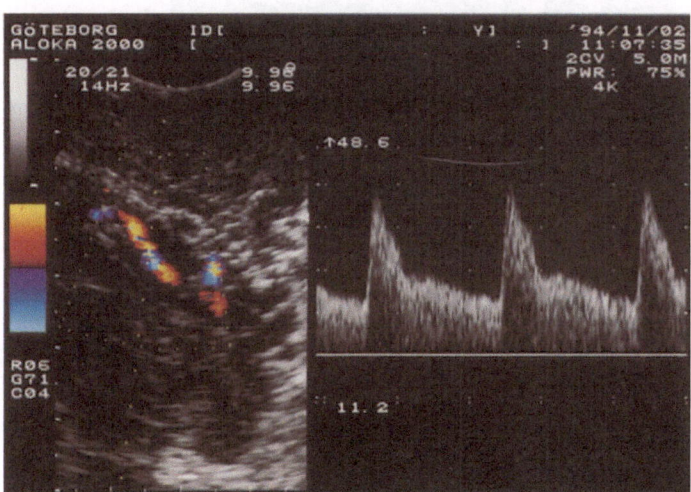

Fig. 3. An example of uterine morphology and flow velocity waveforms demonstrating very low impedance. Pulsatility index (PI), 1.4

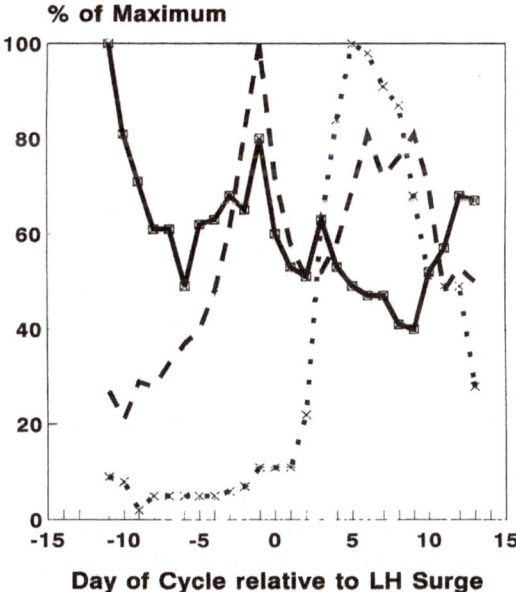

Fig. 4. Daily changes in the pulsatility index (*PI*) and the concentrations of plasma oestradiol and progesterone, relative to the day of peak urinary luteinizing hormone (*LH*)

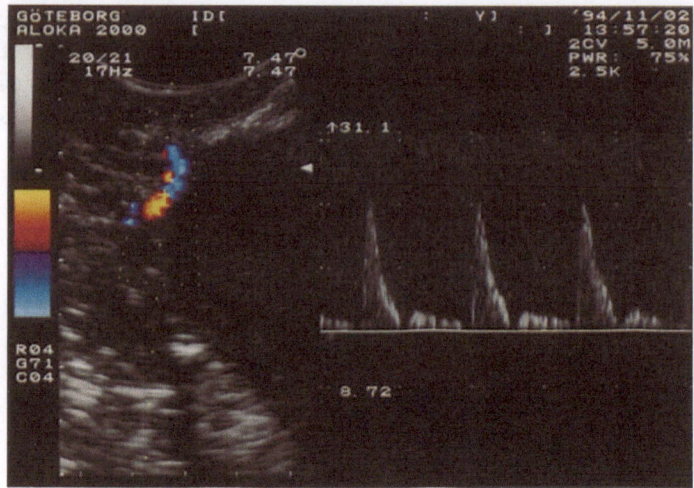

Fig. 5. An example of uterine morphology and flow velocity waveforms demonstrating high impedance. Pulsatility index (PI), 4.6

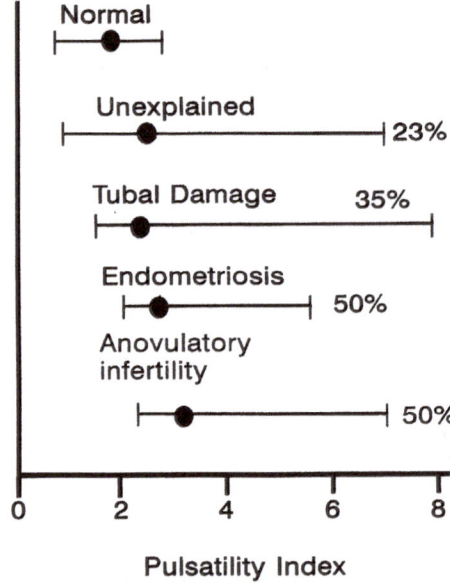

Fig. 6. Median mid-luteal pulsatility index (PI) observed in each category of infertile women compared with fertile women. *Percentages* indicate the proportion of infertile patients in each category with PI values outside the normal range

women with each of the four causes of infertility that were outside the normal PI range. This study [14] was the first report to demonstrate in patients with various causes of female infertility a significant deviation from normal in the impedance to uterine blood flow in the mid-luteal phase, which is the physiological time of implantation of the embryo.

A possible explanation for the increased PI values seen in patients with tubal damage or endometriosis is that the scarring and inflammation associated with these conditions may inhibit the increase in uterine perfusion that would normally occur in the mid-luteal phase in response to physiological endocrine changes. In the case of patients with anovulatory infertility, the most likely explanation for the raised PI is the subnormal hormonal levels on day 21 of the menstrual cycle.

The patients with unexplained infertility are a particularly interesting group. Although they had normal ovarian function and a normal pelvis on laparoscopic assessment, 23% had PI values outside the normal PI range seen in the fertile women. This supports the notion previously reported [5] that decreased uterine artery perfusion might be a cause of unexplained infertility. It is possible that the mechanism mediating this increased uterine impedance may be an attenuation in the uterine arterial response to the circulating ovarian hormones.

This study demonstrates that the uterine artery impedance is significantly increased in women with different causes of infertility compared with women with normal fertility. It provides preliminary evidence in support of abnormal uterine perfusion being a contributory factor to unexplained infertility. Further studies are needed to determine whether ovarian stimulation with gonadotrophin therapy in the subset of infertile patients who have an abnormal mid-luteal uterine artery PI may improve fertility by normalizing uterine artery blood flow at the time of implantation.

Transvaginal Colour Doppler of the Artificial Cycle

In order to assess the effect that quantifying changes in uterine perfusion might have on uterine receptivity, 82 women were selected who had at least three good-quality embryos available for transfer into the uterine cavity in an IVF attempt [13]. Shortly before the embryo transfer, the uterine artery FVW were recorded from both uterine arteries. These were analyzed by the PI, and the outcome of the cycle was compared with the PI values. The concentration of serum E_2 and the mean uterine arterial PI on the day of ET are related to the treatment outcome (i.e. pregnancy or no pregnancy) in Fig. 7. There was no significant correlation between the concentration of serum E_2 and the mean uterine arterial PI in either the women who became pregnant (correlation coefficient r, 0.001) or those who did not (r, −0.088).

There was a significant difference ($p < 0.007$) in the mean uterine PI between those who became pregnant and those who did not. The PI was divided arbitrarily into three ranges (low, 1.00–1.99; medium, 2.00–2.99; and high, 3.0+). A probability of conception of 0.47 was achieved with PI values between 2.00 and 2.99. Nineteen women (23.2%) had a PI value greater than 3.00, and none became pregnant. The pregnancy rate (PR) was 44.4% in the 63 women who had a PI value of less than 3.00. There was no significant difference in the mean (±SD) numbers of embryos transferred between the two groups. The zero implantation rate associ-

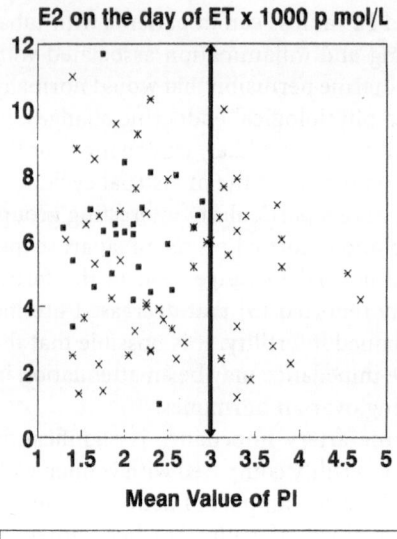

Fig. 7. Mean uterine arterial pulsatility index (*PI*) and serum oestradiol concentration on the day of embryo transfer (*ET*) related to treatment outcome

˟ **Not Pregnant = 54**   • **Pregnant = 28**

ated with a mean PI greater 3.00 was highly significant ($p < 0.001$, Fisher's exact test). If a mean PI value of 3.00 was taken as the upper limit for the transfer of embryos, then the sensitivity of the test for predicting a non-receptive uterus would be 35.2%, the specificity 100%, and the predictive value of a positive scan result 100%.

The results of this study show that measurement of the mean uterine arterial PI is a good method of assessing uterine receptivity during the treatment of infertility by IVF and ET. A mean PI greater than 3.0 prior to the transfer of the embryos could predict up to 35% of failures to become pregnant. No previous method has been published that claims to predict the failure of embryos to implant with this degree of accuracy.

Discussion

Endovaginal colour Doppler is safe; the spacial peak temporal average (SPTA) power output of the machine, for all modalities, is less than 65 mW/cm^2, which is well within the highest limit recommended by the Bioeffects Committee of the American Institute for Ultrasound in Medicine for use in Obstetrics [1]. The procedure is easy to perform and provides rapid results without the need for an endometrial biopsy, which may cause trauma and bleeding at the implantation site with a potential reduction in the chance of pregnancy.

I suggest that the use of this new technique could lead to a significant overall improvement in the success rate of IVF and ET. If uterine conditions were found to be suboptimal, then the embryos could be cryopreserved for transfer in a subsequent cycle (natural or induced) in which uterine receptivity was more appropriate.

Furthermore, preliminary data by Goswmay et al. [5] show that uterine blood perfusion can be improved by the administration of E_2. It appears that optimal uterine receptivity for implantation of an embryo corresponds (using our technique and equipment) to a mean PI of 2.00–2.99. The results of studies with animals have provided a possible explanation why the lowest uterine arterial impedance on the day of ET does not lead to maximal uterine receptivity. For example, it has been shown that a pharmacological dose of E_2 is required to produce maximal uterine artery blood flow in castrated sheep and that peak flow is only maintained for a short period of time [8].

The study on the day of ET has demonstrated that endovaginal blood flow imaging and the use of the PI could have an important role in medically assisted conception and might theoretically improve the PR to almost 50% per ET. Conversely, a group of women has been identified with optimal uterine receptivity (PI, 2.00–2.99) who are at a high risk of developing a multiple pregnancy after ET. Accordingly, it is suggested that under the circumstances a maximum of two good-quality embryos should be transferred.

I believe it is evident that some form of assessment of uterine receptivity will be a significant step forward in infertility management, in particular as related to IVF and ET. It is my opinion that vaginal colour Doppler will be superior to a pure imaging technique, as it can be used as a parameter for monitoring an improvement in receptivity within a treatment cycle. I have observed that prolongation of the follicular (unopposed oestrogen) phase of a down-regulated cycle by oestradiol supplementation at a higher dose than 6 mg results in a lowering of the PI (unpublished observations). Perhaps measurement of the PI can be useful as a monitoring tool to determine the length of oestrogenic stimulation required before optimal conditions for implantation are reached. However, the effectiveness of this approach would require confirmation by a further study. Prospective controlled clinical trials are required to assess the value of these new procedures.

References

1. AIUM (1988) American Institute of Ultrasound in Medicine Bioeffects Report. J Ultrasound Med 7: S1–S38
2. Beier Hellwig K, Sterzik K, Bonn B, Beier HM (1989) Contribution to the physiology and pathology of endometrial receptivity: the determination of protein patterns in human uterine secretions. Hum Reprod 4: 115–120
3. Edwards RG, Craft I (1990) Development of assisted conception. Br Med Bull 46: 565–579
4. Gonen Y, Casper RF, Jacobson W, Blankier J (1989) Endometrial thickness and growth during ovarian stimulation: a possible predictor of implantation in in vitro fertilization. Fertil Steril 52: 446–450
5. Goswamy RK, Williams G, Steptoe PC (1988) Decreased uterine perfusion – a cause of infertility. Hum Reprod 3: 955–959
6. Goswamy RK, Steptoe PC (1988) Doppler ultrasound studies of the uterine artery in spontaneous ovarian cycles. Hum Reprod 3: 721–726

 7. Graf MJ, Reyniak JV, Battle Mutter P, Laufer N (1988) Histologic evaluation of the luteal phase in women following follicle aspiration for oocyte retrieval. Fertil Steril 49: 616–619
 8. Greiss FCJ, Rose JC, Kute TE, Kelly RT, Winkler LS (1986) Temporal and receptor correlates of the estrogen response in sheep. Am J Obstet Gynecol 154: 831–838
 9. Paulson RJ, Sauer MV, Lobo RA (1990) Factors affecting embryo implantation after human in vitro fertilization: a hypothesis. Am J Obstet Gynecol 163: 2020-2023
10. Queenan JT, O'Brien GD, Bains LM, Simpson J, Collins WP, Campbell S (1980) Ultra-sound scanning of ovaries to detect ovulation in women. Fertil Steril 34: 99–105
11. Rogers PA, Milne BJ, Trounson AO (1986) A model to show human uterine receptivity and embryo viability following ovarian stimulation for in vitro fertilization. J In Vitro Fert Embryo Transf 3: 93–98
12. Scholtes MC, Wladimiroff JW, van Rijen HJ, Hop WC (1989) Uterine and ovarian flow velocity waveforms in the normal menstrual cycle: a transvaginal Doppler study. Fertil Steril 52: 981–985
13. Steer CV, Campbell S, Tan SL, Crayford T, Mills C, Mason BA, Collins WP (1992) The use of transvaginal color flow imaging after in vitro fertilization to identify optimum uterine conditions before embryo transfer. Fertil Steril 57: 372–376
14. Steer CV, Tan SL, Mason BA, Campbell S (1994) Midluteal-phase vaginal color Doppler assessment of uterine artery impedance in a subfertile population. Fertil Steril 61: 53–58
15. Tan SL, Steer C, Royston P, Rizk B, Mason BA, Campbell S (1990) Conception rates and IVF. Lancet 335: 299
16. Tan SL, Royston P, Campbell S, Jacobs HS, Betts J, Mason B, Edwards RG (1992) Cumulative conception and livebirth rates after in-vitro fertilisation. Lancet 339: 1390–1394
17. Taylor KJ, Burns PN, Wells PN, Conway DI, Hull MG (1985) Ultrasound Doppler flow studies of the ovarian and uterine arteries. Br J Obstet Gynaecol 92: 240–246
18. Taylor KJ, Burns PN (1985) Duplex Doppler scanning in the pelvis and abdomen. Ultrasound Med Biol 11: 643–658
19. Welker BG, Gembruch U, Diedrich K, Al Hasani S, Krebs D (1989) Transvaginal sonography of the endometrium during ovum pickup in stimulated cycles for in vitro fertilization. J Ultrasound Med 8: 549–553

Uterine and Endometrial Pathology

A.C. Fleischer, T.H. Bourne, J.A. Cullinan, and D.M. Kepple

Introduction

Transvaginal colour Doppler ultrasonography facilitates the study of the uterine vasculature in a number of both physiological and pathological conditions. The main uterine artery can be clearly identified and is often best visualised just lateral to the supravaginal portion of the cervix. The uterine arteries give off arcuate branches which in turn form a circumferential pattern within the interface between the outer and middle layers of the myometrium. At right angles to the arcuate vessels run the radial arteries. These penetrate the endometrium, where they end as spiral arterioles. In some pathological conditions, this ordered vascular pattern may be disrupted. In others, vasodilatation of existing vessels may occur, or new vessels develop as a result of angiogenesis.

The main applications of transvaginal colour Doppler ultrasonography in patients with uterine disorders include:

1. Assisting in the characterisation of endometrial pathology in either symptomatic or asymptomatic postmenopausal women
2. The evaluation of hormone and drug effects on the uterus
3. The assessment of uterine perfusion before and after medical treatment for fibromyomata

This chapter will attempt to discuss these potential applications and try to establish what role transvaginal colour Doppler may have for practising clinicians. Transvaginal colour Doppler ultrasonography depicts the main uterine as well as the arcuate vessels that course within the outer and middle layers of the myometrium. These vessels are arranged in a spoke-wheel configuration and define the boundary between the middle and outer layer of the myometrium [9]. It is more difficult to see vessels more distal to the arcuates such as the radial and spiral arteries in the normal non-pregnant state. However, in certain circumstances, such as under the influence of exogenous hormones, these vessels dilate and may be clearly seen.

Endometrial Disorders Including Cancer

About 30 000 new cases of endometrial cancer are reported in the United States each year. Uterine bleeding is the most frequent initial sign of this disease and at present demands invasive investigation (i.e. endometrial biopsy). However, less than 10% of women with post-menopausal bleeding have endometrial cancer. A less invasive technique than diagnostic biopsy that also has a high detection rate and low false-positive rate would be of value. If this test could detect cancers at an early stage in asymptomatic women, then the number of women cured by surgery alone might be increased, and the morbidity and mortality from the disease reduced. This would be particularly relevant for women at increased risk of developing endometrial abnormalities, such as those taking unopposed oestrogens or tamoxifen therapy [12]. There are now good data to suggest that the measurements of endometrial thickness made using transvaginal ultrasonography can have both high positive and negative predictive values for malignancy. An endometrium that measures greater than 8.0 mm from one myometrial – endometrial interface to another [21] is highly likely to be associated with significant endometrial pathology. There is, however, a significant false-positive rate.

Uterine vascularity is another consideration, and the characteristic flow velocity waveforms that can be obtained from the uterine artery have been described. Recent reports have suggested that transvaginal colour Doppler can be used to reproducibly measure impedance to blood flow in these vessels [1, 25]. As described above, the uterine arteries can be identified in the longitudinal plane slightly lateral to the supravaginal portion of the cervix (Fig. 1). Colour Doppler enables the main branch to be reliably identified and then sampled using pulsed Doppler. This should be carried out once the probe has been angled to obtain the maximum colour intensity from the vessel in question. Using the pulsatility index (PI), a one-way analysis of variance of replicate data from 20 women has given coefficients of variation of the order of 10% for both uterine arteries.

Bourne et al. [3] measured impedance to blood flow in the uterine arteries as well as endometrial thickness in women with postmenopausal bleeding both with and without cancer, as well as women taking hormone replacement therapy and those thought to have a normal uterus taking no drug therapy. Data from this study suggests that, in the presence of malignant tissue, the impedance to uterine artery blood flow is reduced significantly when compared to control groups. In all cases of endometrial carcinoma, the uterine artery PI measured less than 1.8. Impedance to blood flow in the uterine arteries increases with years from the menopause, and so these results cannot be explained by differences in patient age. It may be that this difference can be accounted for by the presence of neovascularisation in the endometrial cavity or possibly because these women are inherently more sensitive to the action of endogenous oestrogens. This may predispose them to the development of endometrial carcinoma as well as being associated with a decreased impedance to flow in the uterine arteries secondary to vasodilation. Data from the same group of women also revealed significant differences in endometrial thickness between the different groups of pathology. Using colour Doppler, the false-positive rate of the B-mode ultrasound-based test was reduced, whilst maintaining sensitivity. If colour Doppler is used to interrogate the endometrium in such cases, angiogenesis can be demonstrated as areas of colour superimposed on the B-mode grey-scale image and the sensitivity of the technique

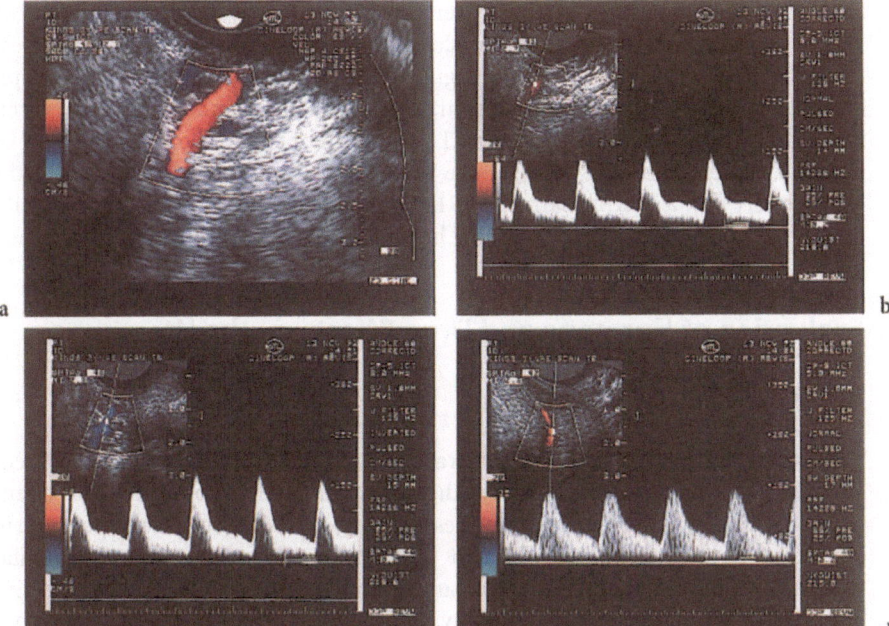

Fig. 1. a The uterine artery visualised at the supravaginal portion of the cervix. **b,c** A pulsed Doppler range gate has been placed sequentially over each uterine artery generating typical flow velocity waveforms. Note the relatively high velocity, low-impedance flow. This is because of the presence of a fibroid in the uterus. **d** The main artery supplying this fibroid has also been examined by pulsed Doppler; the flow velocity waveform is characteristically of low impedance and high velocity

may be enhanced. Perhaps the area where colour Doppler may have most value would be in examining the uterus in cases where the endometrium is thickened to search for areas of angiogenesis. An interesting further observation in this study was that there was a marked reduction in blood flow impedance within the uterine arteries of women taking hormone replacement therapy, a point that will be discussed later in this chapter.

Other workers have also reported vascular changes in the presence of uterine cancer using colour Doppler. In one report, two cases of endometrial cancer were examined, and resistance index (RI) values from the periphery of the endometrial echo were 0.26 and 0.31, respectively [16]. Hata et al. [13] examined ten women with endometrial cancer and found areas of low impedance blood flow in all cases (PI, 0.535 ± 0.158); in patients with uterine myomata, the intra-tumoural blood flow impedance was 0.679 ± 0.131. Our experience of uterine fibroids is that they are characterised by a low-impedance, but high-velocity blood flow picture. Attempts have been made to characterise uterine tumours using transvaginal colour Doppler [17]. Intra-tumoural blood flow was looked for in 291 benign and 17 malignant uterine tumours. The RI value was 0.58 ± 0.12 SD in cases of uterine myomata, and 0.34 ± 0.03 in cases of endometrial carcinoma. The authors conclude that transvaginal colour Doppler can be used help discriminate between benign and malignant uterine tumours and that an intra-tumoural RI value of less than 0.40 should be regarded as malignant and between 0.40 and 0.50 as suspicious. In general, the ultrasound appearances of myomata and endometrial carcinoma are distinct and quite different. To what extent colour Doppler will ever be necessary to discriminate between the two is uncertain. The observation in the same report that a uterine sarcoma (RI, 0.31) had significantly lower impedance blood flow than benign myomata may have more practical clinical implications.

Evaluation of Hormone and Drug Effects on the Uterus

Hormone Replacement Therapy

Following the observation that there was a decreased PI in the uterine arteries of women taking hormone replacement therapy, attempts have been made to quantify this effect. In a subsequent study, oestrogen was shown to reduce impedance to blood flow in the uterine artery by 50% [2]. If extrapolated to the general vasculature, this would have obvious implications with regard to the cardioprotective effect of oestrogen replacement therapy. The changes in uterine artery impedance occurred rapidly. A protein related to the oestradiol receptor has been identified in the intima of major vessels [22], and it is possible that oestrogens affect arterial status through a conventional sex hormone receptor mechanism. The addition of progestogens appear to partially reverse this drop in impedance, although not to pre-treatment levels [14]; this takes effect within 36 h of starting progestogen therapy, suggesting that the mechanism is also receptor mediated [18]. A particularly interesting observation in of the study by Hillard et al. [14] was that the response to exogenous oestrogens was proportional to the number of years since the menopause. If this is confirmed, there may be cardiovascular benefit from oestrogen administration even in very elderly women, as they may still have a significant vascular response to therapy. Selecting progestogens that have the least effect on the vasodilatation brought about by oestrogen therapy may be of great importance if the beneficial effects of hormone replacement therapy are to be maximised; such a choice may be investigated with the use of transvaginal colour Doppler. These data were later supported by that of de Ziegler et al. [26]. In six women with either idiopathic premature ovarian failure or ovarian failure secondary to chemotherapy, uterine artery blood flow was assessed before and during oestrogen therapy. The PI before treatment was 5.2 ± 0.4 (mean ± SEM), dropping to 1.3 ± 0.3 when taking exogenous oestrogens. Studies of other vessels have now shown similar changes in response to oestrogen therapy [23]. Doppler ultrasonography of the aorta has demonstrated that oestrogens increase both stroke volume and flow acceleration. These are thought to reflect a combination of inotropism and vasodilatation. Changes in uterine artery response to exogenous oestrogens seem to act as a model for what is happening in the general vasculature. Transvaginal colour Doppler can therefore be used to assess the effect of hormone replacement therapy on the circulation and on the uterine arteries in particular.

Tamoxifen

It has been proposed that tamoxifen be given to apparently healthy women at increased risk of breast cancer [24]; however, it may be necessary to monitor the endometrium of such patients at regular intervals. Tamoxifen has been shown to provide effective treatment for women with all stages of breast cancer. There are also associated physiological benefits that include a fall in circulating cholesterol concentration and the maintenance of bone density in the lumbar spine. However, these benefits derive from the oestrogenic action that tamoxifen has on tissues other than the breast. It is this possible oestrogen agonist activity that has given rise to concern regarding the effect this drug might have on the endometrium. There have been several reports of the development of endometrial cancer associated with the use of tamoxifen therapy [8, 11, 20]. However, the real risk has been hard to evaluate, given that both breast and endometrial cancer share both hyperoestrogenic and genetic risk factors. In order to evaluate this risk, data from randomised controlled trials are needed [6]. A recent study examined the endometrium of women taking part in a randomised breast cancer prevention trial. The women in the trial received either 20 mg tamoxifen/day or placebo. A total of 25% of women taking tamoxifen had histological evidence of atypical hyperplasia or polyp formation, compared to 4% in the placebo group [15]. In all cases of significant histological abnormality, the endometrial thickness was greater than 8.0 mm and was often cystic in appearance (Fig. 2). Furthermore, the uterine artery PI for all the polyps and cases of atypical hyperplasia was less than 1.8. In view of

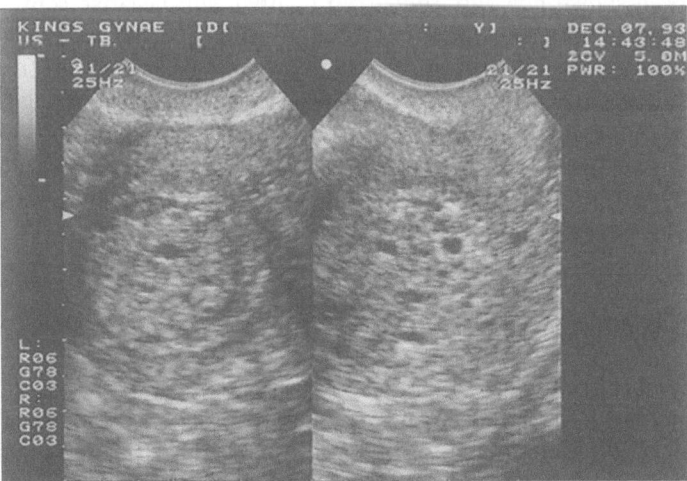

Fig. 2. A thick cystic endometrium typical of a woman taking tamoxifen therapy

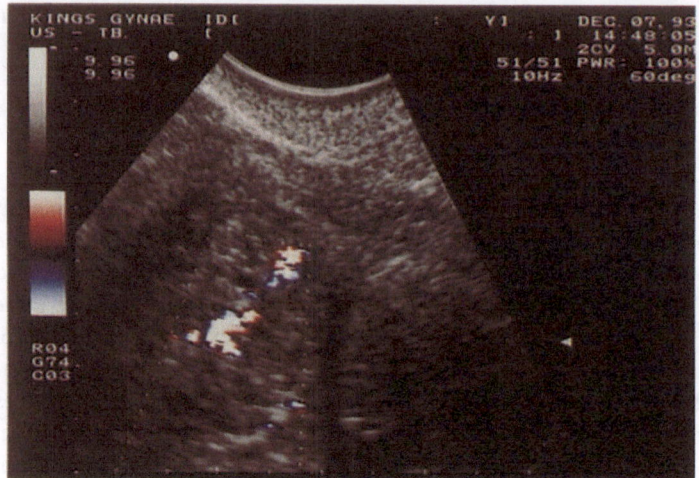

Fig. 3. Thick endometrium of a woman receiving tamoxifen therapy. Colour Doppler has demonstrated an area of blood flow within the cavity. Pulsed Doppler showed a low-impedance waveform. Histology revealed an endometrial carcinoma

the lower dose of drug used in this study, it is difficult to ignore this clear evidence of the association between tamoxifen therapy and the development of endometrial lesions. This study suggests that the presence of thick endometrium (>8.0 mm) in women taking tamoxifen is frequently associated with a significant endometrial abnormality and should be investigated further. In our experience, the finding of a thickened endometrium in this context, which has a vascular pattern consistent with angiogenesis, has a high predictive value for the presence of carcinoma (Fig. 3).

It has also been shown how ultrasound can be used with negative contrast media to demonstrate endometrial lesions associated with the use of tamoxifen therapy [4]. The instillation of sterile saline into the endometrial cavity will help visualise polyps that are often difficult to diagnose even with hysteroscopy (Fig. 4). The use of such negative contrast media should always be considered when investigating the pre- or post-menopausal endometrium. New advances in ultrasound technology in the form of three-dimensional imaging may enable us to characterise these lesions even more accurately.

Gonadotrophin-Releasing Hormone Agonists

Uterine fibroids are frequently found in gynaecological practice and have traditionally been treated by hysterectomy or myomectomy. However, in 1983 Filicori et al. [10] reported that the administration of a gonadotrophin-releasing hormone (GnRH) analogue reduced the size of uterine fibroids. Later, Matta et al. [19] used a pulsed Doppler system to demonstrate that GnRH analogues also reduced blood

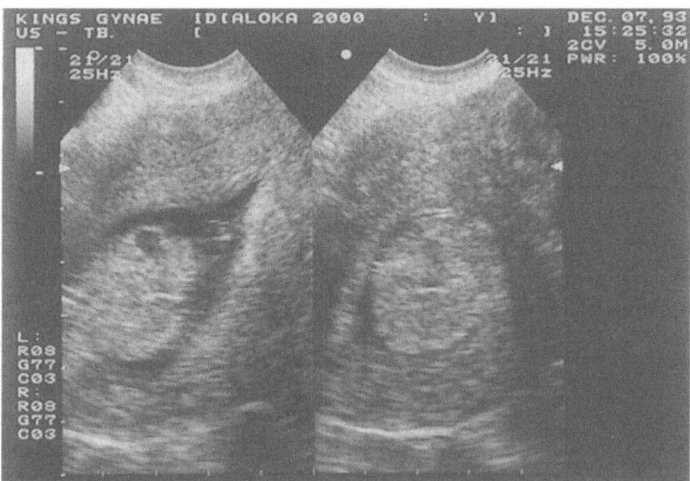

Fig. 4. The endometrial cavity of a woman taking tamoxifen therapy. Sterile saline has been injected into the cavity to reveal a large fleshy endometrial polyp. Subsequent histology revealed areas of focal atypical hyperplasia

flow to fibroids. Generally, a main feeder vessel to a fibroid can be identified around its pseudocapsule and will have a relatively low impedance, high-velocity blood flow pattern. It is tempting to speculate whether there is any association between the vascularity of a particular fibroid and the severity of symptoms experienced by the patient. More recently, Creighton et al. [7] examined a series of fibroids using transvaginal colour Doppler before and after treatment with a GnRH analogue. A median reduction in fibroid size of 52% was noted after just 1 month. A non-linear relationship demonstrated that fibroids with a volume of less than 100 ml are least likely to benefit from down-regulation. There was also a tendency for the median PI in the uterine and main fibroid artery to increase during treatment. There was a corresponding decrease in peak systolic velocity in the same vessels (a mean reduction of 32% and 45%, respectively, after 2 months). This study demonstrated how transvaginal colour Doppler can be used to optimise the use of drugs in gynaecology. It is clear that there is a maximal reduction in both fibroid size and vascularity after just 2 months of treatment with a GnRH agonist.

Conclusion

B-Mode ultrasound imaging provides many answers to the evaluation of the pre and postmenopausal uterus. For example, the endometrial thickness and echogenicity enable the presence or absence of significant pathology to be assessed in the majority of cases. The use of negative contrast agents introduced into the cavity may further enhance diagnostic confidence and be of particular value in the recognition of polyps. Colour Doppler may have a role in identifying characteristic blood flow patterns associated with angiogenesis within the endometrium and may aid in the recognition of the degree of myometrial invasion.

However, there are currently no published data that offer convincing evidence that the addition of colour Doppler to B-mode imaging is necessary for most gynaecologists. It adds to the diagnostic picture, but it is not essential. Where colour Doppler is of great interest is the study of physiological processes and the effects of exogenous drugs and hormones on blood vessels. In this context transvaginal colour Doppler may act almost as a biological assay of end-organ response. This application, alongside the further investigation of vascular changes in both benign and malignant uterine disorders, will make transvaginal colour Doppler an exciting research tool for some time to come.

References

1. Bourne TH, Campbell S, Whitehead MI, Royston P, Steer CV, Collins WP (1990) Detection of endometrial cancer in postmenopausal women by transvaginal ultrasonography and colour flow imaging. Br Med J 301: 369
2. Bourne TH, Hillard T, Whitehead MI, Crook D, Campbell S (1990) Evidence for a rapid effect of oestrogens on the arterial status of postmenopausal women. Lancet 335: 1470–1471
3. Bourne TH, Campbell S, Steer CV, Royston P, Whitehead MI, Collins WP (1991) Detection of endometrial cancer by transvaginal ultrasonography with colour flow imaging and blood flow analysis: a preliminary report. Gynecol Oncol 40: 253–259
4. Bourne TH, Lawton F, Leather A, Granberg S, Campbell S, Collins WP (1994) Use of intracavity saline instillation and transvaginal ultrasonography to detect a tamoxifen associated endometrial polyp. Ultrasound Obstet Gynecol 4: 73–75
5. Bourne TH, Kedar RP, Collins WP, Cosgrove DO, Campbell S, Ashley SE, Powles TJ (1995) Screening for uterine abnormalities in postmenopausal women participating in a randomised trial of tamoxifen for the prevention of breast cancer. Lancet (submitted)
6. Craig Jordan V (1993) How safe is tamoxifen? Only randomised controlled trials can decide. Br Med J 307: 1371–1372
7. Creighton S, Bourne TH, Lawton FG, Crayford T, Vyas S, Campbell S, Collins WP (1994) Use of transvaginal ultrasonography with color Doppler imaging to determine an appropriate treatment regimen for uterine fibroids before surgery: a preliminary report. Ultrasound Obstet Gynecol 4: 494–498
8. Cohen I, Shapiro H, Haller M (1993) Endometrial changes in postmenopausal women treated with tamoxifen for breast cancer. Br J Obstet Gynaecol 100: 567–570
9. Farrer-Brown G, Beilby JOW, Tarbit MH (1990) The blood supply to the uterus. 1. Arterial vasculature. J Obstet Gynaecol Br 77: 673–681
10. Filicori M, Hall DA, Loughlin JS, Vale W, Crowley WF (1983) A conservative approach to the management of uterine leiomyomata: pituitary desensitisation by a luteinising hormone releasing hormone analogue. Am J Obstets Gynecol 147: 726–727
11. Fornander T et al (1989) Adjuvant tamoxifen therapy in early breast cancer: occurrence of new primary cancers. Lancet i: 117–120
12. Hardell L (1989) Tamoxifen as a risk factor for carcinoma of the corpus uteri. Lancet 60: 126–131
13. Hata K, Makihara K, Hata T, Takahashi K, Kitao M (1991) Transvaginal color Doppler imaging for haemodynamic assessment of tumors in the reproductive tract. Int J Gynecol Obstet 36: 301–308

14. Hillard TC, Bourne TH, Crayford T, Collins WP, Campbell S, Whitehead MI (1993) Differential effects of transdermal estradiol and sequential progestagens on impedance to flow within the uterine arteries of postmenopausal women. Fertil Steril 58: 959–963
15. Kedar RP, Bourne TH, Powles TJ, Collins WP, Cosgrove DO, Campbell S (1994) Effects of Tamoxifen on the uterus and ovaries of women involved in a randomised breast cancer prevention trial. Lancet 343: 34–28
16. Kurjak A, Zalud I, Jurkovic D, Alfirovic Z, Miljan M (1989) Transvaginal color flow Doppler for the assessment of pelvic circulation. Acta Obstet Gynecol Scand 68: 131–135
17. Kurjak A, Zalud I (1991) The characterisation of uterine tumours by transvaginal colour Doppler. Ultrasound Obstet Gynecol 1: 50–52
18. Marsh MS, Bourne TH, Whitehead MI, Collins WP, Campbell S (1994) The temporal effect of progesterone on uterine artery pulsatility index in postmenopausal women receiving sequential hormone replacement therapy. Fertil Steril 62: 771–774
19. Matta WHM, Stabile I, Shaw RW, Campbell S (1988) Doppler assessment of uterine blood flow change in patients with fibroids receiving the gonadotrophin releasing hormone buserelin. Fertil Steril 49: 1083–1085
20. Neven P (1993) Tamoxifen and endometrial lesions. Lancet ii: 452
21. Osmers R, Volksen M, Schauer A (1990) Vaginosonography for early detection of endometrial carcinoma. Lancet i: 1569–1571
22. Padwick ML, Whitehead MI, Coffer A, King RJB (1989) Demonstration of estrogen receptor related protein in female tissues. In: Studd JWW, Whitehead MI (eds) The menopause. Blackwell, Oxford, pp 227–233
23. Pines A, Fisman EZ, Levo Y, Averbuch M, Lidor A, Drory Y, Finkelstein A, Hetman-Peri M, Moshkowitz M, Ben-Ari E, Ayalon D (1991) The effects of hormone replacement therapy in normal postmenopausal women: measurements of Doppler-derived parameters of aortic flow. Am J Obstet Gynecol 164: 806–812
24. Powles TJ, Hardy SE, Ashley SE, Farrington GM, Cosgrove D, Davey JB, Dowsett M, McKinna JA, Nash AG, Sinnett HD, Tillyer CR, Treleaven JG (1989) A pilot trial to evaluate the acute toxicity and feasibility of tamoxifen for prevention of breast cancer. Br J Cancer 60: 126–131
25. Steer CW, Campbell S, Pampligione J, Kingsland CR, Mason BA, Collins WP (1990) transvaginal colour flow imaging of the uterine arteries during the ovarian and menstrual cycles. Human Reprod 5: 391
26. de Ziegler D, Bessis R, Frydman R (1991) Vascular resistance of uterine arteries: physiological effects of estradiol and progesterone. Fertil Steril 55: 775–777

Investigation of the Utero-Placental Circulation

E. JAUNIAUX, D. JURKOVIC, and S. CAMPBELL

Introduction

Until recently Doppler ultrasound studies of the utero-placental circulation have been limited to the late second and third trimesters of pregnancy. The introduction of transvaginal transducers has enabled studies of the utero-placental and fetal circulations in the first trimester.

Transabdominal pelvic ultrasound examination is most successful when the patient's bladder is full. However, bladder filling displaces pelvic organs backwards, increasing the distance between the Doppler probe and the vessels of interest, thus only permitting the use of low-pulse repetition frequencies. Furthermore, a distended bladder may also cause alteration in blood flow in small arteries and occasionally causes significant patient discomfort, limiting the examination time. For all these reasons the accuracy and reproducibility of transabdominal Doppler studies in early pregnancy has been unsatisfactory. By using the transvaginal route, most of these technical problems are eliminated. The probe can be located close to the vessel under investigation and the optimal pulse repetition frequencies can be selected.

After 12 weeks of gestation, the pregnant uterus is large enough to be examined transabdominally without the need for a full bladder. If the gestational sac is located in the upper third of the uterus, investigation of the placental circulations by the transvaginal route may be difficult and the transabdominal route is usually preferred.

In the present chapter, we have reviewed the role of transvaginal colour Doppler in the investigation of the uteroplacental circulation in normal and complicated pregnancies.

Correlation of Doppler Features and Anatomical Changes During the Development of Utero-Placental Circulation

Fundamental anatomical and physiological differences exist between the environment of the developing embryo and that of the developing fetus. These differences are so great that they justify the statement that the first trimester pregnancy is a different biological entity from the second or third trimester pregnancy [17]. Classically, when the blastocyst starts to implant, a number of endometrial vessels

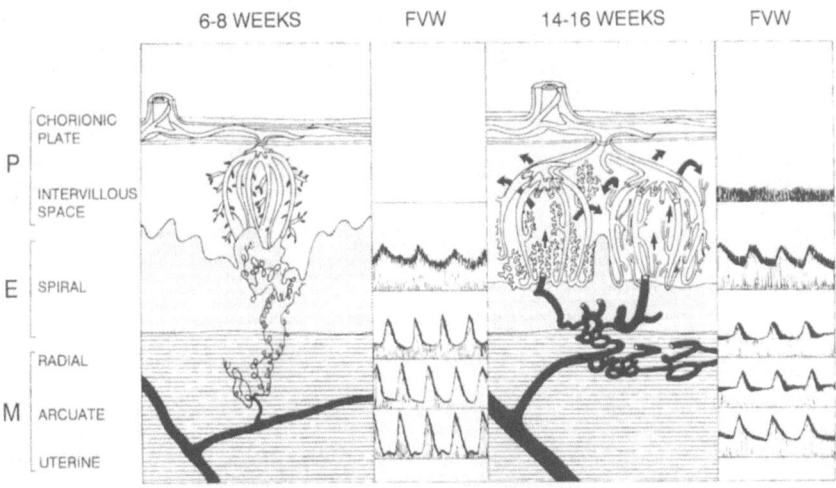

Fig. 1. Various flow velocity waveforms (*FVW*) obtained from the utero-placental circulations at 8 and 16 weeks of gestation, respectively. (Modified from [15])

are opened by the phagocytic activity of trophoblast; maternal blood enters the intervillous space, establishing the utero-placental circulation. This theory has been challenged by the results of Hustin and Schaaps, who showed that during the first trimester of pregnancy the growing embryo and its placenta are separated from the maternal uterine circulation by trophoblastic plugs that obliterate the tip of the utero-placental arteries (see chapter by Hustin on "Vascular Physiology and Physiopathology of Early Pregnancy"). Around 12 weeks of gestation, these plugs are progressively dislocated, allowing maternal blood to flow freely in the intervillous space.

The various branches of the uterine circulation can be differentiated by means of colour Doppler imaging (Fig. 1). The overall Doppler features correlate well with both classical and modern anatomic findings [24]. In non-pregnant patients and during the first half of normal pregnancies, blood flow velocity waveforms from the main uterine arteries are characterized by a well-defined proto-diastolic "notch" (Fig. 2). By contrast, the transformed spiral arteries are characterized by low-impedance turbulent flow. Recognition of this typical flow pattern during the entire pregnancy is useful in the early diagnosis of ectopic pregnancy (see chapter by Jurkovic et al. on "Transvaginal Colour Doppler in Ectopic Pregnancies"). The expression "trophoblastic flow", which has been used in early studies to describe spiral artery blood flow is inaccurate and should be abandoned. Flow velocity waveforms generated by the intervillous circulation can be detected during the second and third trimesters inside the placental tissue (Fig. 3). This flow is continuous, non-pulsatile and is not found before 12 weeks in normal pregnancies [13–16].

Studies using either continuous wave or pulsed Doppler have demonstrated a progressive decrease in downstream resistance to blood flow in the uterine artery

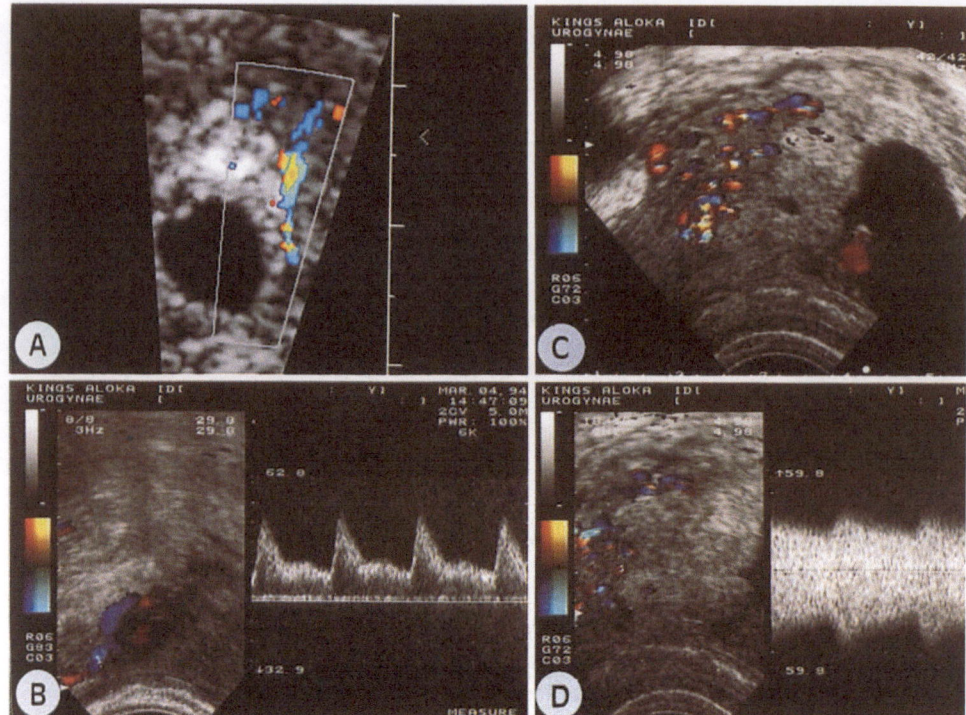

Fig. 2A–D. Transvaginal colour Doppler mapping of a terminal portion of the uteroplacental circulation at 5 + 6 weeks of gestation (**A**) and spectral analysis of blood velocity waveforms obtained from the main uterine artery at 9 + 2 weeks (**B**). C Colour mapping of the placental bed. D Spectral analysis of blood velocity waveforms obtained from a spiral artery at 10 + 1 weeks. Note the absence of colour signal inside the placental mass

during the first trimester of pregnancy [5, 11, 21, 27]. This decrease continues during the second and the third trimesters and can be observed in all segments of the uterine circulation (Fig. 4). A decrease in the resistance and pulsatility indices from the main uterine artery towards the spiral arteries can also be demonstrated at different stages of pregnancy [14, 15].

Transvaginal colour Doppler examination of the uterine artery allows accurate estimation of the angle between the vessels and the pulsed Doppler beam [15, 21]. Doppler measurements performed at an angle of insolation of less than 10° eliminate angle-dependant errors in maximum and mean velocity calculations. These data demonstrate an exponential and significant increase in the mean peak systolic velocity of the main uterine artery around 13 weeks of gestation (Fig. 5), which corresponds to the time of establishment of the utero-placental circulation. A relationship between the establishment of continous intervillous flow and an abrupt increase in the mean uterine artery velocity has been reported [15, 16], possibly corresponding to the dislocation of the tropho-

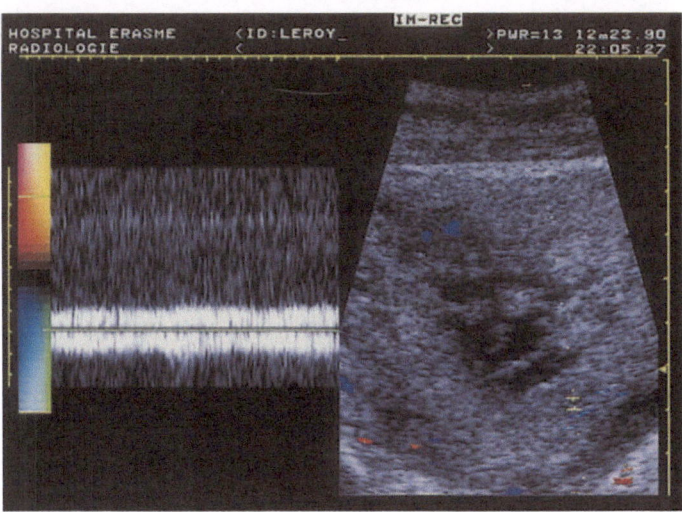

Fig. 3. Transabdominal colour Doppler mapping and spectral analysis demonstrating continuous blood flow with a venous pattern (i.e. intervillous flow) at 13 + 1 weeks of gestation

blastic plugs, which allows uninhibited blood flow circulation in the entire intervillous space.

Relationship Between Doppler Features, Uterine Anatomy and Maternal Endocrinology in Early Pregnancy

Implantation and placental development in primates are associated with complex changes in the uterine wall constituents [24]. The most striking of these transformations is observed soon after implantation at the level of the spiral arteries. Their architecture is disrupted, with the loss of myocytes from the media and the internal elastic lamina as they develop into the utero-placental arteries [23]. As a result, there is a progressive fall in the downstream resistance to uterine blood flow, as shown by Doppler studies. In human pregnancy, uterine vascular changes have been closely related to trophoblast infiltration of the placental bed and the concomitant erosion of the spiral arteries [23]. However, in some animal species, such as horses, pigs and all ruminants, no trophoblastic infiltration or destruction of the maternal tissue occurs and the conceptus is adequately supplied by maternal blood [4]. Furthermore, Doppler studies have shown that the reduction in uterine vascular resistance starts during the luteal phase before implantation and that no difference can be found in uterine blood flow from normal intra-uterine pregnancies and from ectopic pregnancies where placentation is distant from the uterine cavity. This suggests that changes in uterine blood flow in early pregnancy are not exclusively dependent on trophoblast infiltration and that other factors must act to modulate uterine blood flow.

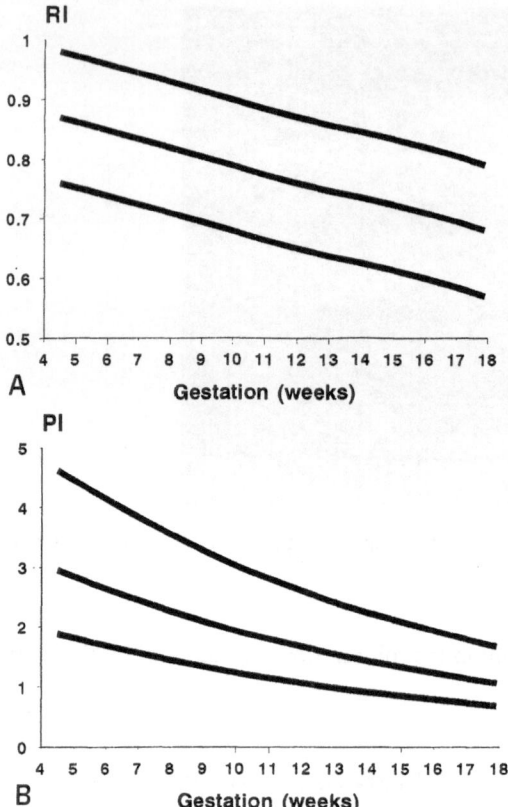

Fig. 4A,B. Reference ranges (mean and 95% confidence interval) of the resistance index (*RI*; **A**) and pulsatility index (*PI*; **B**) in the main uterine artery with gestational age

Estradiol was found to influence the uterine resistance index in early pregnancy [18] and its effect may be modulated by maternal relaxin serum levels [19]. Estrogens and progestagens are known to have an antagonistic effect on the general vasculature and it is likely that steroid effects are determined more by changes in the estrogen to progestagen ratio than by the level of each individual hormone (see chapter by Bourne et al. on "Ovulation and the Periovulatory Follicle"). These findings are in agreement with the results of experiments on animals which have shown that direct intra-arterial uterine infusion of E_2 produces a dramatic increase in uterine blood flow in both pregnant and non-pregnant uterine vascular bed, while progesterone partially inhibits the vascular effect of E_2 [1]. Furthermore, recent Doppler studies of the internal carotid and uterine artery of post-menopausal women receiving hormone replacement therapy have shown that at physiological levels E_2 decreases the resistance to flow as measured by pulsatility indices in both circulations and that this is partially reversed by progestagen [6, 8]. The rapid fall in resistance with gestation as demonstrated by angle-independent Doppler indices is probably secondary to the combined action of several factors, including hormonal effects and trophoblast infiltration.

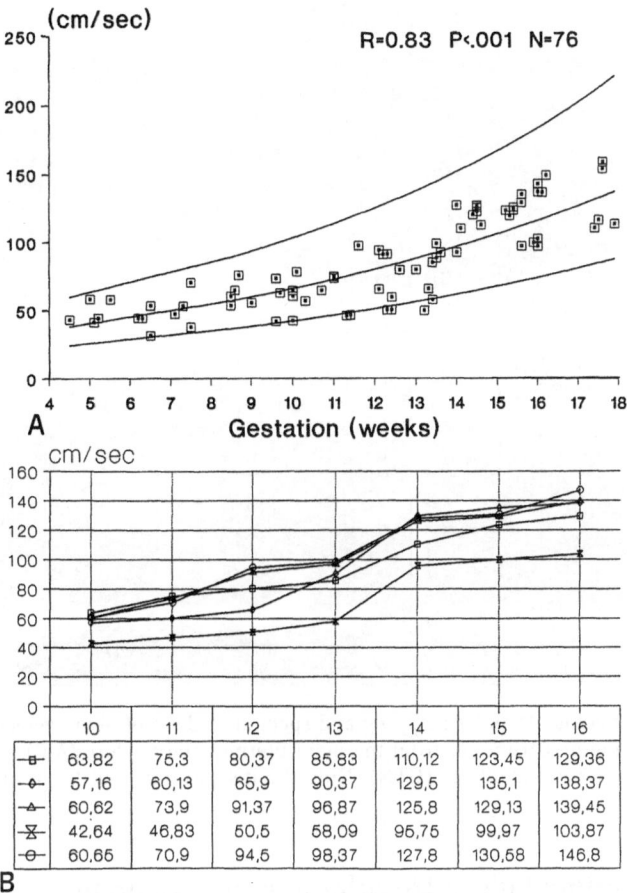

Fig. 5. **A** Individual values and reference ranges (mean and 95% confidence interval) of the peak systolic velocity (cm/s) in the main uterine artery with gestational age. **B** Individual mean values by gestational week of the peak systolic velocity (cm/s) in the main uterine artery measured longitudinally in five normal pregnancies between 10 and 16 weeks of gestation. (Modified from [15])

	10	11	12	13	14	15	16
-□-	63,82	75,3	80,37	85,83	110,12	123,45	129,36
-◆-	57,16	60,13	65,9	90,37	129,5	135,1	138,37
-▲-	60,62	73,9	91,37	96,87	125,8	129,13	139,45
-✕-	42,64	46,83	50,5	58,09	95,75	99,97	103,87
-⊖-	60,65	70,9	94,5	98,37	127,8	130,58	146,8

There is now increasing evidence that the generation of nitric oxide (NO) from L-arginine by the vascular endothelium plays a key role in the control of vascular tone [25]. Intravenous glyceryl trinitrate (GTN), a donor of NO in vivo, given in the first trimester can mimic the physiological alteration of the uterine artery flow velocity waveform seen with advancing gestation (Fig. 6), suggesting that the adaptation of the maternal cardiovascular system to pregnancy is due to increased production of endogenous NO [25]. It is likely that pre-eclampsia is associated with a defect in this mechanism. Incompletely modified vessels as found in early pregnancy and in those at high risk of pre-eclampsia are more likely to react favourably to GTN than those which have lost their media, because nitrates act on the vascular smooth muscle to cause vasodilatation [25].

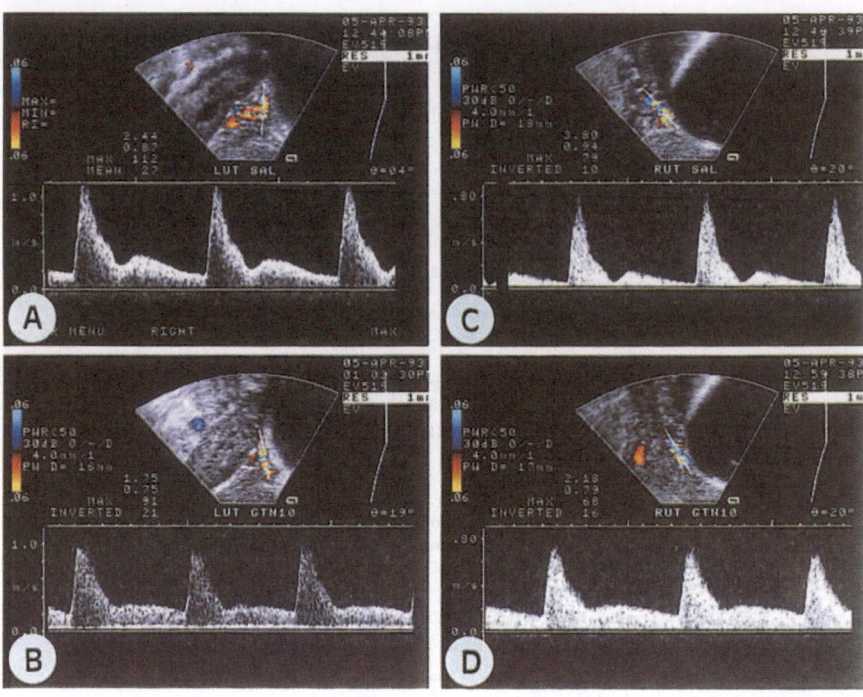

Fig. 6A–D. Transvaginal colour Doppler mapping and spectral analysis of blood velocity waveforms obtained in the first trimester from the main uterine artery before (**A,C**) and after (**B,D**) intravenous glyceryl trinitrate (GTN). Note the disappearance of the proto-diastolic notch

Safety of Transvaginal Colour Doppler in Early Pregnancy

Tissue heating is the main concern when ultrasound equipment is used during pregnancy. Animal studies indicate that cell death, interruption of proliferative activity and vascular damage can be found in embryonic tissues when the temperature increases 1.5°C above the normal baseline [29]. This may result in both developmental defects and abortion. However, marked differences in basal body temperature between species make it difficult to extrapolate animal data to the human embryo.

The surface temperature of ultrasound transducers increases by about 0.5°C/mW per cm² after 5 min in the air [7], thus commercial Doppler equipment should be considered as a potential heat source. The increase in temperature generated by a transducer will be mainly absorbed by the surrounding tissues. With endovaginal probes, the short distance between the transducer and embryo makes heating from the transducer more likely. The potential for heating is further increased by the use of high-frequency transducers (5–10 MHz). Modern endovaginal transducers usually offer three diagnostic facilities: B-mode, pulsed Doppler and colour Doppler. In terms of ultrasonic power intensity output, the pulsed Doppler mode is most likely to expose the embryo to potentially harmful levels [7]. The risk to the embryo can be substantially reduced if the length of the pulsed Doppler examination is reduced to a minimum.

The ability to visualize vessels of interest by colour Doppler simplifies blood flow studies and shortens the use of pulsed Doppler to just a few seconds. At the same time a reliable and easy identification of the vessels prevents unnecessary exposure of the embryo and other tissues to the "wandering" pulsed Doppler beam. It is also important to be familiar with output parameters of the ultrasound equipment. The parameter that is most commonly used is spatial peak temporal average intensity and it should be less than 100 mW/cm^2 for studies of the embryonic or fetal circulation [29]. Other important parameters should be obtained from the manufacturer, such as the focal length, scan length, centre frequency, source diameter and transducer surface temperature. Heating hazards can also be reduced by cooling the ultrasound probe between the examination in antiseptic solution and switching off the equipment.

Predicting Abnormal Utero-Placental Development

Transvaginal colour Doppler now facilitates the detection of flow velocity waveforms from small vessels such as from the terminal part of the utero-placental circulation. This has led to much enthusiasm on the part of clinicians interested in predicting early and late pregnancy complications related to an abnormal placentation.

Two recent histological studies have demonstrated that in cases of spontaneous abortion there is an inadequate placentation and, in particular, a defective transformation of the spiral arteries, which seems not to be linked with chromosomal anomalies [9, 22]. Reduced trophoblastic penetration into the decidua and into the spiral arteries has also been demonstrated in most cases of spontaneous abortions, while in normal pregnancies physiological changes are always present [9]. Furthermore, the trophoblastic columns are reduced in number and the trophoblastic shell is thinner and discontinuous in pregnancies complicated by anomaly or death of the conceptus. These features are more pronounced in early pregnancies complicated by partial and complete hydatidiform moles [10].

Pathological findings suggest that one of the functions of trophoblastic plugging of spiral arteries is to restrict maternal blood flow into the intervillous space in early pregnancy. An interesting ultrasound feature of complicated pregnancy in the first trimester is the ability to detect, in all cases of missed abortion and in nearly all cases of very early embryomic death, an intervillous flow (Fig. 7) before 12 weeks of gestation [20, 26]. The free entry of maternal blood into the intervillous space at this stage of gestation disrupts the placental shell and may be the mechanical cause of abortion [20]. It remains to be investigated whether these abnormal patterns may be used to diagnose abnormal implantation and predict spontaneous abortion in the first trimester.

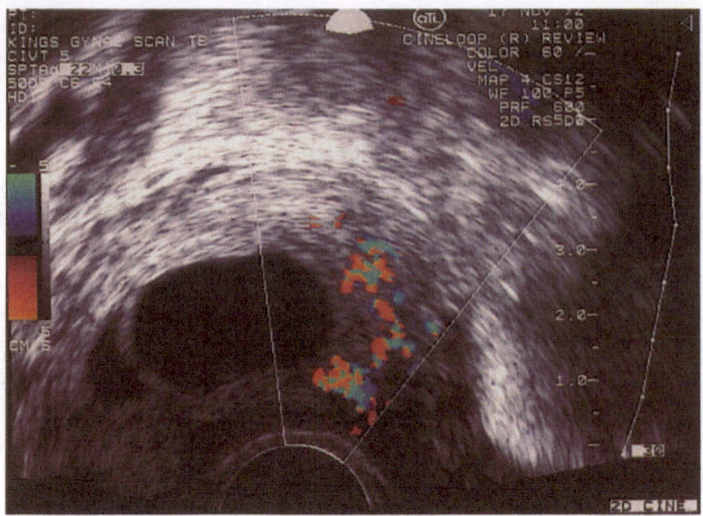

Fig. 7. Intervillous blood flow in an anembryonic pregnancy at 9 weeks of gestation

Authors using abdominal pulsed-wave Doppler equipment to study early pregnancies longitudinally have demonstrated a more marked decrease in the resistance index in pregnancies destined to become abnormal [28]. However, all recent transvaginal Doppler studies in the first trimester have failed to show abnormal blood flow indices in the utero-placental circulation of pregnancies that subsequently ended in complete abortion or in missed abortion [2, 12, 20]. This finding supports the hypothesis that factors other than trophoblastic infiltration of the placental bed regulate the transformation of the spiral arteries. It is suggested that even in cases of missed abortion with or without embryomic remmants, where the trophoblastic infiltration can be significantly reduced, sufficient placental endocrinological activity is maintained to allow the development of a normal utero-placental circulation. Only studies comparing Doppler features with pathological findings will permit a better understanding of the pathophysiology of early pregnancy complications [20].

In 85% of pregnancies, the proto-diastolic notch disappears before 20 weeks of gestation [3]. An increased impedance to flow in the utero-placental circulation at 18–22 weeks and persistent notching predicts the development of pregnancy-induced hypertension and/or intra-uterine growth retardation later in gestation [3]. These abnormal Doppler features have been associated with defective placentation and in particular with reduced or absent trophoblastic invasion and inadequate transformation of the spiral arteries. These findings strongly support the hypothesis that spontaneous abortion and pregnancy-induced hypertension are part of the same pathological process, which involves a failure, a delay or an insufficiency of physiological changes associated with haemochorial placentation [9, 22]. New studies are currently being performed to evaluate the ability of transvaginal colour Doppler imaging in early pregnancy to predict which patients will subsequently develop preeclampsia, intra-uterine growth retardation or placental abruptio.

Acknowledgement   This work was supported by the David and Alia VanBuuren Foundation (ULB).

References

1. Anderson SG, Hackshaw BT, Still JG, Greiss FC (1977) Uterine blood flow and its distribution after chronic estrogen and progesterone administration. Am J Obstet Gynecol 127: 138–142
2. Arduini D, Rizzo G, Romanini C (1991) Doppler ultrasonography in early pregnancy does not predict adverse pregnancy outcome. Ultrasound Obstet Gynecol 1: 180–185
3. Bower S, Schuchter K, Vyas S, Campbell S (1993) The study of uterine artery blood flow to predict IUGR and pregnancy induced hypertension. Obstet Gynecol 82: 78–83
4. Burton GJ (1992) Human and animal models: limitations and comparisons. In: Barnea E, Hustin J, Jauniaux E (eds) The first twelve weeks of gestation. Springer, Berlin Heidelberg New York, pp 469–485
5. Deutinger J, Rudelstorfer R, Bernaschek G (1988) Vaginosonographic velocimetry of both main uterine arteries by visual recognition and pulsed Doppler method during pregnancy. Am J Obstet Gynecol 159: 1072–1076
6. de Ziegler D, Bessis R, Frydman R (1991) Vascular resistance of uterine arteries: physiological effects of estradiol and progesterone. Fertil Steril 55: 775–779
7. Duck FA, Starritt HC, Haar GR (1989) Surface heating of diagnostic ultrasound transducers. Br J Radiol 62: 1005–1013
8. Gangar KF, Vyas S, Whitehead M, Crook D, Meire H, Campbell S (1991) Pulsatility index in internal carotid artery in relation to transdermal oestradiol and time of menopause. Lancet 338: 839–842
9. Hustin J, Jauniaux E, Schaaps JP (1990) Histological study of the materno-embryonic interface in spontaneous abortion. Placenta 11: 477–486
10. Hustin J, Jauniaux E (1992) Morphology and mechanisms of abortion. In: Barnea E, Hustin J, Jauniaux E (eds) The first twelve weeks of gestation. Springer, Berlin Heidelberg New York, pp 469–485
11. Jaffe R, Warsof SL (1991) Transvaginal color Doppler imaging in the assessment of uteroplacental blood flow in the normal first-trimester pregnancy. Am J Obstet Gynecol 164: 781–785
12. Jaffe R, Warsof SL (1992) Color doppler imaging in the assessment of uteroplacental blood flow in abnormal first trimester intrauterine pregnancies: an attempt to define etiologic mechanisms. J Ultrasound Med 11: 41–44
13. Jaffe R, Woods JR (1993) Color Doppler imaging and in vivo assessment of the anatomy and physiology of the early uteroplacental circulation. Fertil Steril 60: 293–297
14. Jauniaux E, Jurkovic D, Campbell S, Kurjak A, Hustin J (1991) Investigation of placental circulations by color Doppler ultrasound. Am J Obstet Gynecol 164: 486–488
15. Jauniaux E, Jurkovic D, Campbell S (1991) In vivo investigations of the anatomy and the physiology of early human placental circulations. Ultrasound Obstet Gynecol 1: 435–445
16. Jauniaux E, Jurkovic D, Campbell S, Hustin J (1992) Doppler ultrasonographic features of the developing placental circulations: correlation with anatomic findings. Am J Obstet Gynecol 166: 585–587
17. Jauniaux E (1992) Contribution to the study of early pregnancy patho-physiology. PhD thesis, Free University of Brussels

18. Jauniaux E, Jurkovic D, Delogne-Desnoek J, Meuris S (1992) Influence of human chorionic gonadotropin, oestradiol and progesterone on uteroplacental and corpus luteum blood flow in normal early pregnancy. Hum Reprod 7: 1467–1473
19. Jauniaux E, Johnson MR, Jurkovic D, Ramsay B, Campbell S, Meuris S (1994) The role of relaxin in the development of the uteroplacental circulation in early pregnancy. Obstet Gynecol 84: 338–342
20. Jauniaux E, Zaidi J, Jurkovic D, Campbell S, Hustin J (1994) Comparision of Colour Doppler features and pathological findings in complicated early pregnancy. Hum Reprod 9: 2432–2437
21. Jauniaux E, Jurkovic D, Campbell S (1995) In vivo investigation of the placental circulation by Doppler echography. Placenta (in press)
22. Khong TY, Liddell HS, Robertson WB (1987) Defective haemochorial placentation as a cause of miscarriage. A preliminary study. Br J Obstet Gynaecol 94: 649–655
23. Pijnenborg R, Bland JM, Robertson WB, Brosens I (1983) Uteroplacental arterial changes related to interstitial trophoblast migration in early human pregnancy. Placenta 4: 397–414
24. Ramsey EM, Donner NW (1980) Placental vasculature and circulation. Thieme, Stuttgart
25. Ramsay B, de Belder A, Campbell S, Moncada S, Martin JF (1994) A nitric oxide donor improves uterine artery diastolic blood flow in normal early pregnancy and in women at high risk of pre-eclampsia. Eur J Clin Invest 24: 76–78
26. Schaaps JP, Hustin J (1988) In vivo aspect of the maternal-trophoblastic border during the first trimester of gestation. Trophoblast Res 3: 39–48
27. Schulman H, Fleischer A, Farmakides G, Bracero L, Rochelson B, Grunfeld L (1986) Development of uterine artery compliance as detected by Doppler ultrasound. Am J Obstet Gynecol 155: 1031–1036
28. Stabile I, Bilardo C, Panella M, Campbell S, Grudzinskas JG (1988) Doppler measurements of uterine blood flow in the first trimester of normal and complicated pregnancies. Trophoblast Res 3: 301–307
29. WFUMB Working Group (1990) Geneva report on safety and standardisation in medical ultrasound: issues and recommendations regarding thermal mechanisms for biological effects of ultrasound. World Federation for Ultrasound in Medicine and Biology, Geneva, pp 9–17

Transvaginal Colour Doppler in Trophoblastic Disease

F. Flam

Introduction

The trophoblastic cells forming the outer cell mass of the early blastocyst can be identified as early as 4–5 days after fertilization [8]. A few days later they start to penetrate the uterine mucosa, thus initiating the formation of the placenta. The trophoblastic cells erode the endothelial lining of the maternal vessels, making the exchange of nutrients possible. In addition to invasiveness, the trophoblasts of early pregnancy also display other tumour-like properties, such as explosive proliferation and evasion of immuno-surveillance [11]. The trophoblast does not invade beyond the endometrium and the mechanisms behind this strict control are not fully understood. However, there are data supporting the view that extra-embryonic growth factors and receptor interactions are involved and controlled via local stimulatory loops [7]. In invasive mole and choriocarcinoma, the control mechanisms are no longer in effect. In invasive mole, placental tissue invades the myometrium and metastases can also develop. Since the villi cannot be distinguished microscopically from villi in hydatidiform mole, this is not a true cancer. Invasive mole can only occur following a molar pregnancy.

Choriocarcinoma is a true cancer and can develop from a molar pregnancy as well as from other pregnancy events. These two entities are grouped together under the heading GTT (gestational trophoblastic tumors). Persistent disease following a hydatidiform mole may thus come either as invasive mole or as choriocarcinoma. Since chemotherapy is highly effective in the treatment of persistent disease, there is seldom need for hysterectomy. The nature of the disease, invasive mole or choriocarcinoma, will thus be unknown. In the pre-chemotherapy era (before the mid-1950s), hysterectomies were performed in GTT, and from these reports it has been estimated that around 3% of molar patients will eventually suffer from choriocarcinoma [2]. The rest that are treated will then be cases of invasive mole. The American policy has traditionally been to treat between 20%–30% of the molar patients, while centres in Europe have adopted a more strict policy treating only about 10% of these patients. In our centre 7% of the patients with hydatidiform mole will subsequently receive chemotherapy [6].

Hydatidiform Mole

The sonographic appearance of a molar pregnancy is a very characteristic one. The uterus is enlarged with a hyperechoic endometrial complex, which may contain multiple hypoechoic and anechoic spaces. In complete hydatidiform mole, no fetus is visualized. Sonography for this diagnosis was already being used as early as 1963 [10]. Doppler ultrasound is of little additional value in establishing the diagnosis. There are rare cases of local placental abnormalities, such as angiomas, that may simulate cystic villi. The use of colour Doppler will quickly settle this question.

It would be tempting to apply colour Doppler at the stage of diagnosing the molar pregnancy to determine the likelihood of subsequent persistent GTT. However, in characteristic cases the massive amount of placental tissue seems to fill up the uterus, offering a very thin lining of myometrium to study. In addition, these fast-growing, large moles are the ones in the highest risk group and the ones that should really be studied with respect to myometrial invasion. The question of whether the mole is already invasive at this stage or whether it eventually becomes so is unsettled. It may well be that moles at the stage of diagnosis respect the endometrial–myometrial border.

Tumour Imaging

In the work-up of patients with GTT, it is essential to establish the extent of uterine as well as metastatic disease. It can be argued that the outcome of this investigation will not influence the treatment, since chemotherapy will be initiated in any event. However, as in other tumour investigations, increased knowledge of the tumour will be of importance in several respects. Firstly, the extent and localization of the uterine tumour is of importance, should the decision to perform a dilation and curettage (D&C) be made. Particular care should be taken in performing a D&C if the tumour reaches the serosa. Secondly, hysterectomy is sometimes considered in cases where resistance to chemotherapy has developed. If no tumour has been localized within the uterus, the chances of success with this procedure are small. Thirdly, a negative uterine examination could be a cause for concern. Absence of tumour within the uterus means that the hCG most likely is produced by distant metastases.

In 1955 Borell et al. Performed the first angiographic studies in GTT and demonstrated the value of this method [3]. The morphological features of the tumour vessels were characteristic. The uterine arteries were prominent and hypervascular; pooling and arterio-venous shunting were frequently encountered. Angiography was replaced by real-time sonography at most centres as technical advances were made. Later, imaging methods such as computed tomography and magnetic resonance imaging began to be been applied in GTT, but their value has not been proven to be superior to that of sonography.

Colour Doppler in Gestational Trophoblastic Tumours

In their pioneering work dealing with intra-tumoural blood flow, Shimamoto and colleagues [12] studied one hydatidiform mole and five cases of invasive mole. Since then most reports on the use of colour Doppler and GTT are in the form of

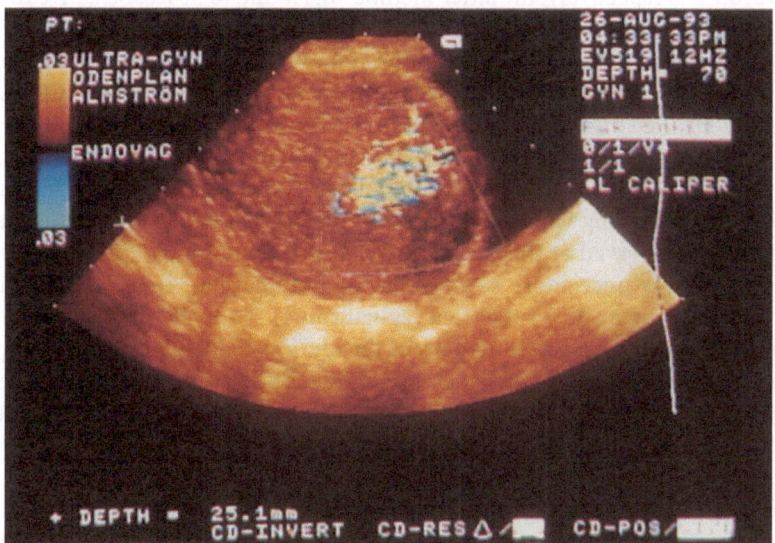

Fig. 1. Sagittal transvaginal sonogram showing neovascularization in the uterus

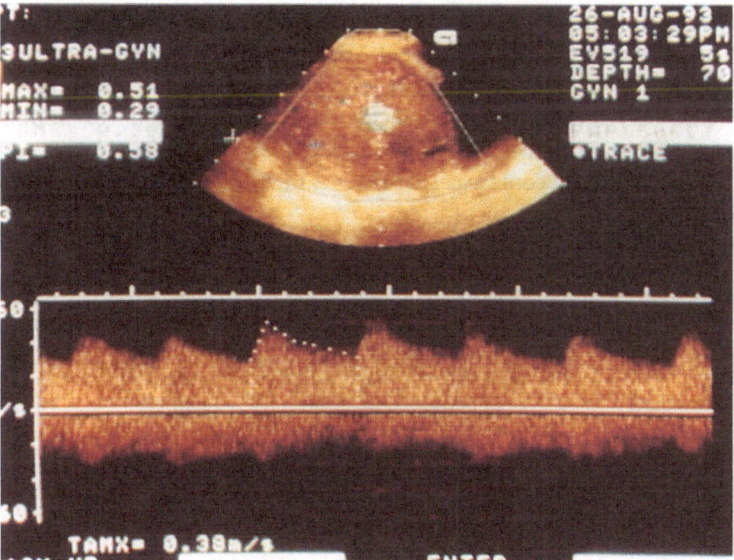

Fig. 2. Sagittal transvaginal sonogram demonstrating blood flow of low resistance

case reports [1, 4]. The main reason for the absence of systematic studies is probably the relative infrequency of GTT.

Following the introduction of TCD, a non-invasive imaging method has evolved that offers more information than B-mode sonographic examinaton. In a study comparing colour Doppler (transabdominal), pelvic angiography and real-time ultrasound, respectively, the latter method was found to be less sensitive than the others in the ten patients thus evaluated [5]. In cases of widespread uterine disease, the diagnosis will be obvious by B-mode imaging alone, but in less advanced cases colour Doppler will be needed in order to provide visual proof of existing tumour. Since the time of the initial study quoted above, angiography at our institution has been replaced by TCD. Fifteen patients were evaluated by TCD and all in all 25 patients with GTN have subsequently been examined (unpublished data). Grey-scale imaging was initially applied in each patient. Abnormal echoes were sometimes observed at this stage. Thereafter, colour Doppler was activated and the uterus was once more scanned in longitudinal and transverse planes (Acuson 128, 5-MHz probe for the transvaginal route). To ensure that the vessels obtained by colour Doppler were actually of the low impedance-type, pulsed Doppler was used to examine tumour vessels at random. The waveforms thus obtained demonstrated characteristic low-impedance, high-velocity patterns. Pulsatility indices were not routinely recorded.

An attempt was made to assess the tumour load. The area of hypervascularization was measured at both planes and a rough estimation of the tumour volume was made. Arbitrarily, a small area was defined as less than 1 cm^3, intermediate as $1-2.5 \text{ cm}^3$ and a large area as greater than 2.5 cm^3. In seven patients (28%), the colour Doppler examination was negative. Two of these patients suffered from choriocarcinoma (antecedent pregnancy other than hydatidiform mole), while five patients had persistent disease. Out of six patients with clear-cut choriocarcinoma, only one patient demonstrated a large area of neovascularization in her uterus (Table 1). It is well known that patients with choriocarcinoma may have widespread metastatic disease with no or minimal uterine tumour. Therefore, absence of colour Doppler signals in patients with choriocarcinoma should not come as a surprise. As mentioned above, five patients

Table 1. Colour Doppler in choriocarcinoma

Patient no.	Colour Doppler area	hCG IU/l	Metastases	Chemotherapy courses
1	Large	220 000	Vagina, lungs	4 single, 7 EMA/Co
2	Intermediate	27 300	–	14 single
3	Small	66 500	–	6 single, 4 EMA/Co
4	Small	4 430	–	9 single
5	Negative	34 500	Brain, lungs	5 EMA/Co
6	Negative	852	Lungs	11 single
Mean		58 900		7.3 single + 2.7 EMA/Co

hCG, human chorionic gonadotrophin.

with persistent disease also demonstrated negative colour Doppler examinations. None of these had metastases. Assuming that choriocarcinoma in persistent disease behaves in much the same way as choriocarcinoma following other pregnancies, a negative colour Doppler finding might be a cause for concern. However, all of these were speedily treated by single-agent drugs. The two highest human chorionic gonadotrophin (hCG) values in this subset of patients were found to be 7300 IU/l and 6000 IU/l. For the patients with persistent disease and a positive colour Doppler examination, there was a rough correlation between the area of neovascularization and the time to reach remission, although statistical significance was not reached. This is much the same as the correlation of the level of hCG to prognosis. This is to be expected since both factors reflect tumour load.

TCD in GTT is easy to apply and offers less pitfalls than other conditions occurring in the pelvic region. In reality, a non-pregnant normal uterus should not give rise to intense colour Doppler signals [9]. Thus the finding of a hyper vascular area associated with high hCG levels is suggestive of persistent GTT. Pulsed Doppler can be used to verify this assumption. It is only rational that TCD in GTT should be easy to perform. The conditions for applying colour Doppler are perfect in such a highly vascularized tissue as the placenta. Therefore, since TCD is particularly easy to perform in GTT, anyone seeing only a couple of cases per year should not refrain from performing this investigation.

References

1. Aoki S, Hata T, Hata K, Senoh D, Miyao J, Takamiya C, Iwanari O, Kitao M (1989) Doppler color flow mapping of an invasive mole. Gynecol Obstet Invest 27: 52–54
2. Bagshawe KD (1969) Choriocarcioma. Arnold, London
3. Borell U, Fernström I, Westman A (1955) The value of pelvic arteriography in the diagnosis of mole and chorionepithelioma. Acta Radiol 44: 378–384
4. Desai RK, Desberg AL (1991) Diagnosis of gestational trophoblastic disease: value of endovaginal color flow Doppler sonography. AJR 157: 787–788
5. Flam F, Lindholm H, Bui TH, Lundström-Lindstedt V (1991) Color Doppler studies in trophoblastic tumors: a preliminary report. Ultrasound Obstet Gynecol 1: 350–353
6. Flam F, Lundström-Lindstedt V, Rutqvist LE (1992) Incidence of gestational trophoblastic disease in the Stockholm County 1975–1988. Eur J Epidemiol 8: 173–177
7. Franklin GC, Holmgren L, Donovan M, Adam G, Walsh C, Pfeifer-Ohlsson S, Ohlsson R (1993) Expression and control of PDGF stimulatory loops in the developing placenta. Troph Res 7: 287–303
8. Hertig AT, Rock J, Adams CE (1956) A description of 34 human ova within the first 17 days of development. Am J Anat 98: 435–459
9. Kurjak A, Zalud I, Jurkovic D, Alfirevic Z, Miljan M (1989) Transvaginal colour Doppler for the assessment of pelvic circulation. Acta Obstet Gynecol Scand 68: 131–135
10. Mac Vicar J, Donald I (1963) Sonar in the diagnosis of early pregnancy and its complications. J Obstet Gynaecol Br Commonw 70: 387–395
11. Ohlsson R (1989) Growth factors, protooncogenes and human placental development. Cell Differ Dev 28: 1–16
12. Shimamoto K, Sakuma S, Ishigaki T, Makino M (1987) Intratumoral blood flow: evaluation with color Doppler echography. Radiology 165: 683–685

III. Ovaries and Fallopian Tubes

Vascular Changes During the Ovarian Cycle

L. VALENTIN

Introduction

The first to publish Doppler measurements of blood flow indices in the uterine and ovarian arteries were Taylor and co-workers [14], who in 1985 compared flow velocity waveforms obtained transabdominally from the iliac, uterine and ovarian arteries with those obtained from the same vessels intra-operatively; they also recorded indices of blood flow from the uterine arteries through the lateral vaginal fornices [14]. Since then a number of reports have been published both using transabdominal and transvaginal Doppler examinations of the uterine and/or ovarian arteries performed longitudinally during the normal menstrual cycle (Table 1). Given the methodological diversity of these studies (see Table 1), it is hardly surprising that they yielded results that differed in many respects. However, some results are common to several of them.

Change in Uterine Artery Waveforms

Values for the blood flow velocity waveform index recorded from the uterine arteries differ considerably from one study to another. For instance, little or no diastolic flow in the uterine arteries was a common finding in one study [4], whereas continuous forward flow in diastole was almost invariably recorded in others [12, 13]. Such discrepancies are probably to be explained by differences in sampling techniques (e.g. transabdominal versus transvaginal) or in the sensitivity of the Doppler ultrasound systems used.

A postovulatory increase in uterine artery impedance to blood flow was reported by five research teams [3, 4, 11–13]. Furthermore, considerably lower values for uterine artery blood flow impedance were recorded in the mid-luteal phase than in the follicular phase of the menstrual cycle in four studies [1, 4, 12, 13]. In only two studies were the results for the dominant and non-dominant uterine artery reported separately; in both studies similar values for pulsatility index were recorded from the dominant and non-dominant uterine artery, even though slightly lower values were obtained from the dominant artery in the mid-luteal phase of the cycle [11, 12].

In our own study on uterine blood circulation during the normal menstrual cycle [12], we examined both uterine arteries lateral to the cervix at the

Table 1. Longitudinal studies on blood flow velocity in the uterine and ovarian arteries during the normal menstrual cycle

Publication	TAS or TVS	CD used?	Doppler frequency (MHZ)	Arteries examined (sampling site)	Cycle days (cds) examined	Results expressed as
Goswamy and Steptoe 1988 [4]	TAS	No	3	Uterine arteries (lateral to cervix)	Not predetermined; twice weekly	S/D ratio, RI, "blood flow classes"
Battaglia et al. 1990 [1]	TAS	Yes	3.5	Uterine arteries (lateral to cervix)	Not predetermined; every 2 days	PI
Steer et al. 1990 [13]	TVS	Yes	6.0	Uterine arteries (lateral to cervix)	Not predetermined; every 3–6 days	PI; % change in PI
Hata et al. 1990 [7]	TAS	Yes	3.5	Ovarian arteries (infundibulo-pelvic ligament or ovarian stroma)	Predetermined; cds 5–7, 11–13, 15–17 and 26–28 (i.e. four per cycle)	PI
Mercé et al. 1992 [9]	TAS	No	3.5	Ovarian arteries (parenchyma adjacent to follicle/corpus luteum)	Not predetermined; every 1–3 days	RI
Bourne et al. 1991 [2]	TVS	Yes	5	Ovarian arteries (wall of dominant follicle/corpus luteum)	Periovulatory period, cds 12–13; every 3–8 h	RI, PI, PSV; % change in PSV
Collins et al. 1991 [3]	TVS	Yes	5	Uterine arteries (sampling site?) Ovarian arteries (wall of dominant follicle/corpus luteum)	Periovulatory, period, cds 12–16; every 3–8 h	PI, PSV
Scholtes et al. 1990 [11]	TVS	No	4.25	Uterine arteries (lateral to cervix) Ovarian arteries (infundibulo-pelvic ligament)	Predetermined; cds 7, 13, 16, 21	PI
Sladkevicius et al. 1993 [12]	TVS	Yes	5	Uterine arteries (lateral to cervix, beneath the endometrium) Ovarian arteries (ovarian hilum, ovarian stroma, wall of largest follicle, wall of corpus luteum)	Predetermined; cds 4, 8, 12, then daily until follicular rupture and 1, 2, 5, 7 and 12 days after follicular rupture	PI, TAMXV

TAS, transabdominal sonography; TVS, transvaginal sonography; CD, colour Doppler; RI, resistance index; PI, pulsatility index; TAMXV, time-averaged maximum velocity; PSV, peak systolic velocity.

level of the internal os and small vessels situated immediately beneath the endometrium ("subendometrium"). Typical Doppler shift spectra from the two sampling sites are shown in Fig. 1. The results of our studies of blood flow velocity in the uterine arteries during the menstrual cycle are presented in Fig. 2. The most striking results were the high values for pulsatility index recorded 2 days after presumed ovulation, and the low values for pulsatility index and high values for time-averaged maximum velocity recorded in the mid- and late-luteal phases.

Change in Ovarian Artery Waveforms

Values for blood flow impedance were much higher when the Doppler signal from ovarian arteries was obtained from the infundibulo-pelvic ligament [7, 11] than when it was obtained from within the ovary itself [9, 12].

Longitudinal studies of ovarian blood flow during the normal menstrual cycle have shown the blood flow impedance of the arteries of the dominant ovary to be lower in the luteal than in the follicular phase and to be lower in the arteries of the dominant than of the non-dominant ovary in the luteal phase of the menstrual cycle [7, 9, 11, 12]. In three studies, little or no change in the values for blood flow

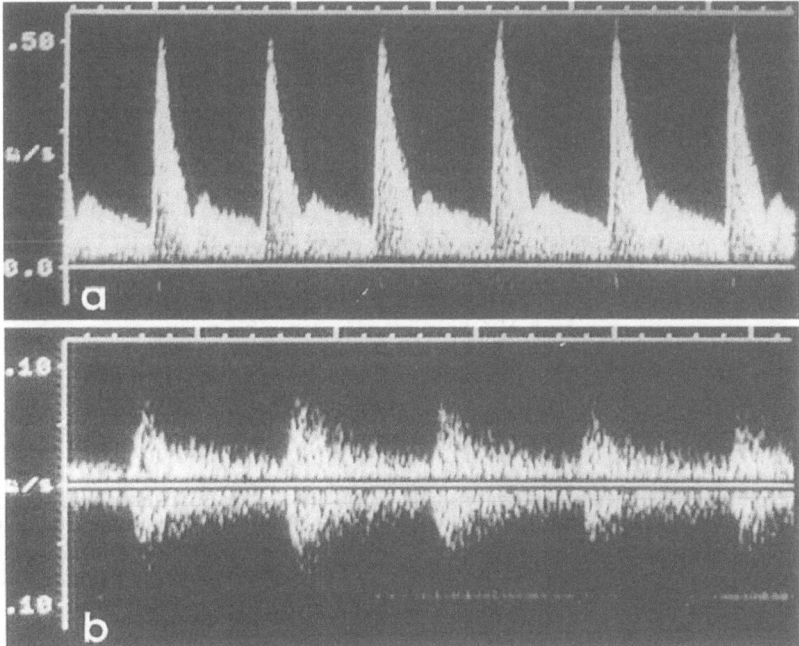

Fig. 1a,b. Typical Doppler shift spectra obtained from the uterine artery (**a**) and from an artery situated immediately beneath the endometrium (**b**). The equipment used was an Acuson 128 XP ultrasound system with a 5-MHz transvaginal probe

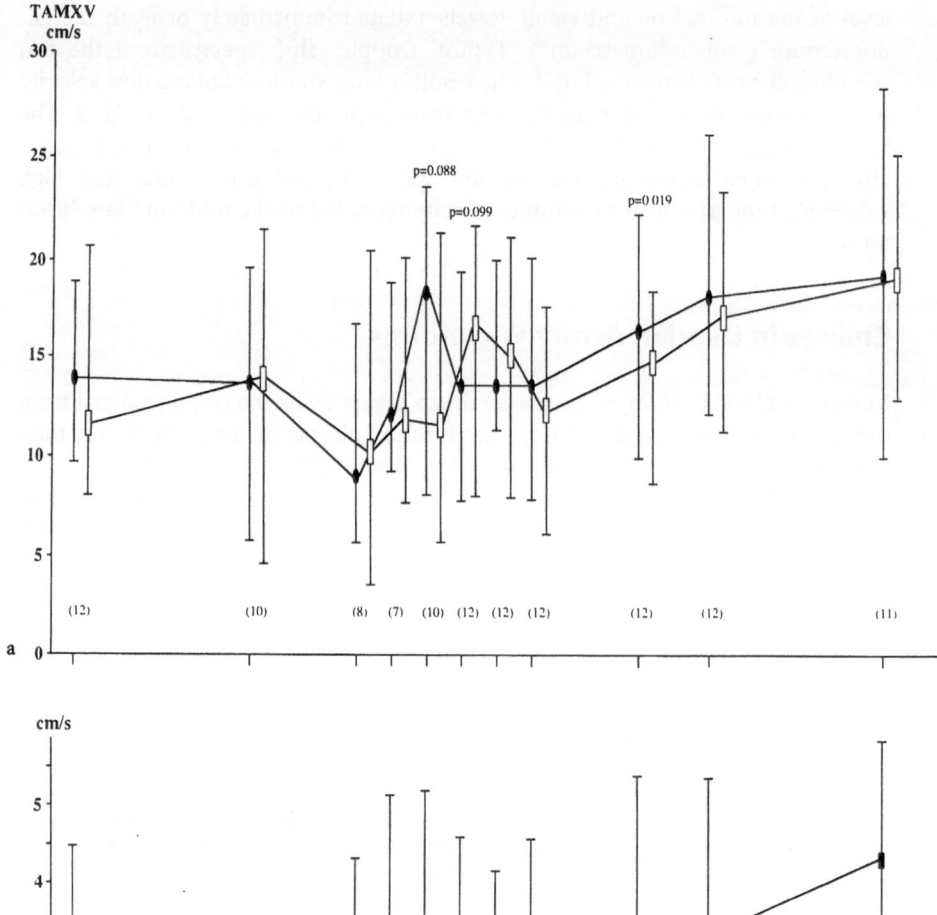

Fig. 2a–d. Time-averaged maximum velocity (*TAMXV*) and pulsatility index (*PI*) in the uterine and subendometrial arteries during the menstrual cycle. **a,c** The uterine arteries. **b,d** The subendometrial arteries. The *filled circles* represent the dominant uterine artery, the *open squares* the non-dominant uterine artery and the *filled squares* the subendometrial arteries. Median, tenth and 90th percentile values are given. The figures in *brackets* denote the number of measurements. The results are expressed in relation to the time of presumed ovulation determined from the ultrasound image, the last day that the dominant follicle was visible on the ultrasound screen being day −1 and the first day that the corpus luteum was visible on the ultrasound screen day 1, etc. Ovulation was presumed to have occurred between the examinations on day −1 and day 1. (Slightly modified from [12]; published with permission from the Parthenon Publishing Company)

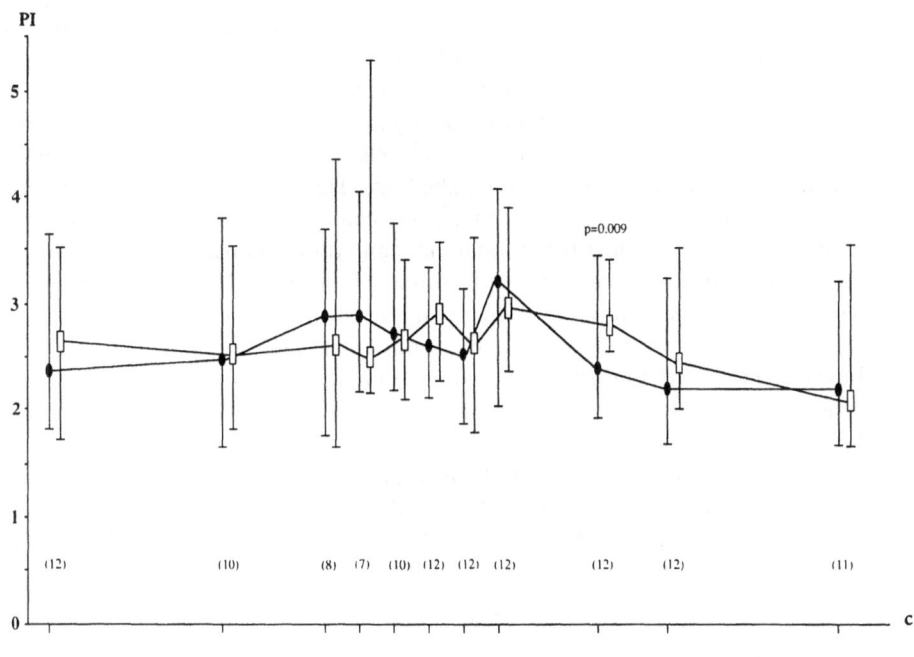

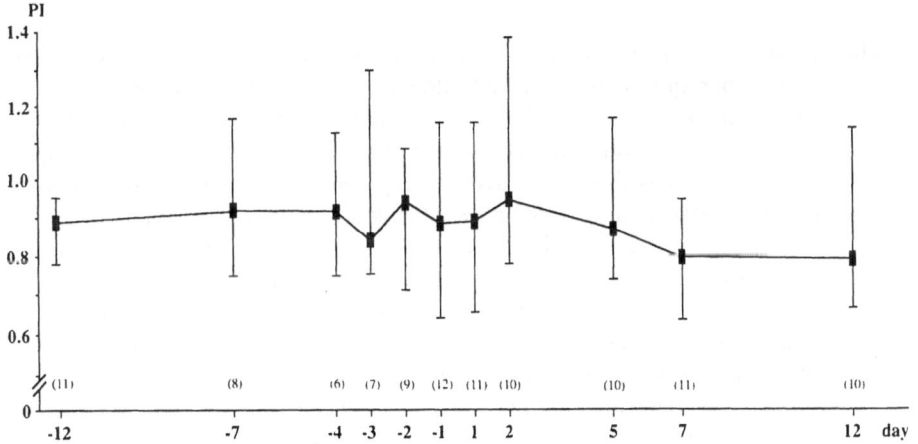

impedance was observed in the arteries of the non-dominant ovary during the menstrual cycle [7, 9, 12].

We have found unequivocal identification of the ovarian artery in the infundibulo-pelvic ligament extremely difficult. In our own study on ovarian blood flow during the menstrual cycle [12], we investigated ovarian circulation by examining arteries in the ovarian hilum (on the surface of the ovary), in the ovarian stroma (any small artery in the ovarian stroma, but not near to the surface or to the largest follicle of the ovary), in the wall of the largest follicle and in the wall of the corpus luteum. Typical Doppler shift spectra from these four sites are shown in Fig. 3, and the results of our blood flow velocity measurements in the ovarian arteries in Fig. 4. The most striking result was the dramatic post-ovulatory increase in time-averaged maximum velocity in the vessels of the dominant ovary. The changes in blood flow velocity in the vessels of the dominant ovary during the menstrual cycle were obvious to the naked eye. The ovary bearing the dominant follicle became successively more intensively coloured (especially the wall of the dominant follicle) 1–2 days before ovulation, and the ovary harbouring the corpus luteum was more intensively coloured, contained more colour spots and was easier to examine than the same ovary before ovulation and than the contralateral ovary. Typical colour Doppler images of the dominant follicle and corpus luteum are shown in Fig. 5. As the intensity of the colour in the colour-coded ultrasound image reflects the intensity-weighted mean velocity of blood in the blood vessels [8], an increase in colour intensity should reflect increased blood velocity (assuming a constant insonation angle and constant settings of the ultrasound system). Our interpretation of the increase in the number of coloured areas in the dominant ovary after ovulation is that an increase in blood flow velocity enabled blood flow to be detected in a greater number of vessels.

Current Development

The findings that, in the vessels of the uterus and dominant ovary, blood flow velocity is higher and the impedance to flow lower in the luteal phase than in the follicular phase of the menstrual cycle may indicate increased blood flow to the uterus and dominant ovary after ovulation; in cerebral vessels the time-averaged maximum velocity was shown to correlate very well with total brain flow, whereas the pulsatility index demonstrated a less strong correlation [5, 6, 10].

Although the colour Doppler image would appear to yield substantial information about the vascularization of an organ, it is difficult to derive an objective measurement that can be used for statistical calculations from the subjective evaluation of the colour Doppler image. New ways of evaluating the information in the colour Doppler image may prove helpful in the future.

Our own research team and that at King's College Hospital in London seem to be the only ones to have studied changes in blood flow velocity (time-averaged maximum velocity and peak systolic velocity, respectively) in the arteries of pelvic organs during the menstrual cycle; both teams found that much more dramatic changes occur in the blood flow velocity than in the impedance indices during the menstrual cycle [2, 3, 12]. The use of blood flow velocity (e.g. time-averaged maximum velocity or peak systolic velocity) to express the results of Doppler measurements in small and/or tortuous vessels might well be questioned. As the angle between the insonating Doppler ultrasound beam and the direction of the blood flow in the blood vessel being examined cannot be determined, it is not possible to measure the true velocity of blood. Although in our own studies, we have always tried to obtain the highest possible Doppler shift, we do not claim to

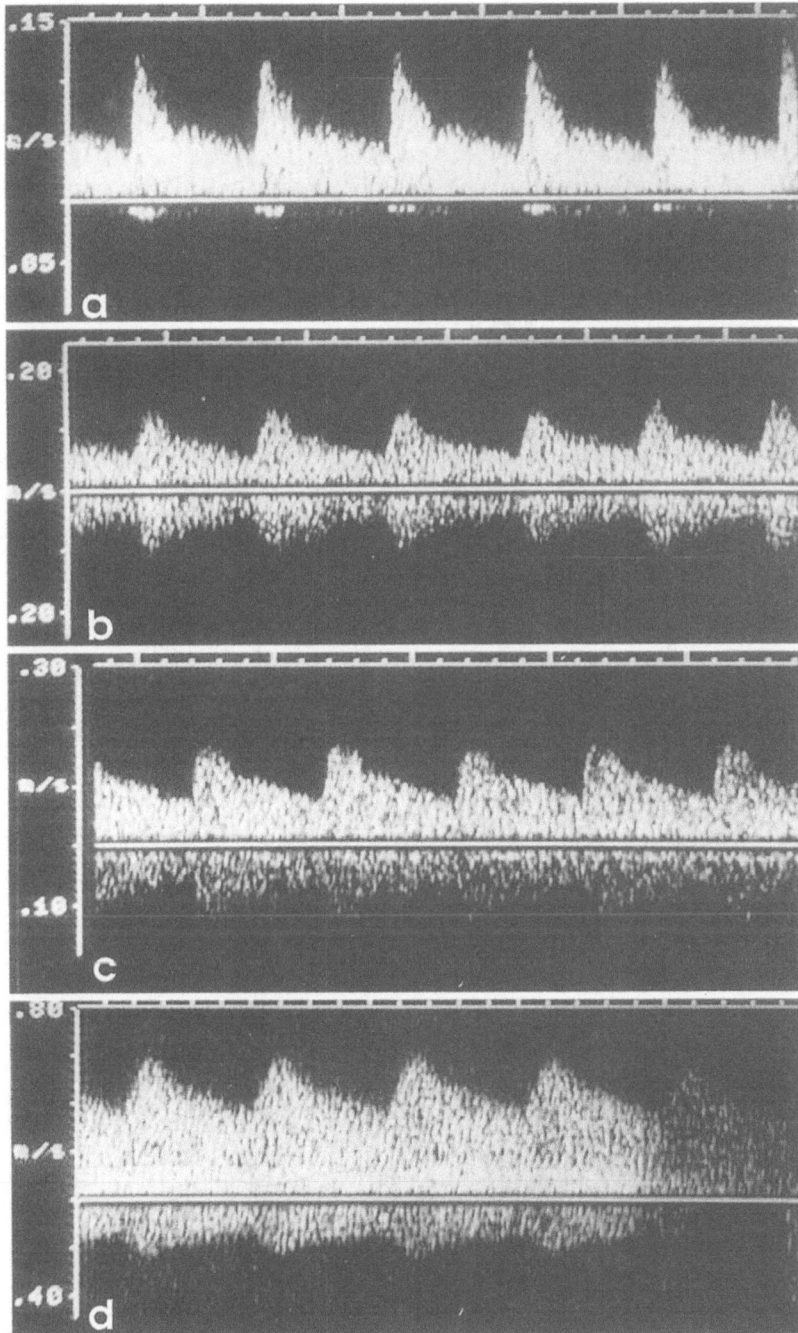

Fig. 3a–d. Typical Doppler shift spectra obtained from arteries in the ovarian hilum (a), ovarian stroma (b), wall of the dominant follicle (c) and wall of the corpus luteum (d). The equipment used was an Acuson 128 XP ultrasound system with a 5-MHz transvaginal probe

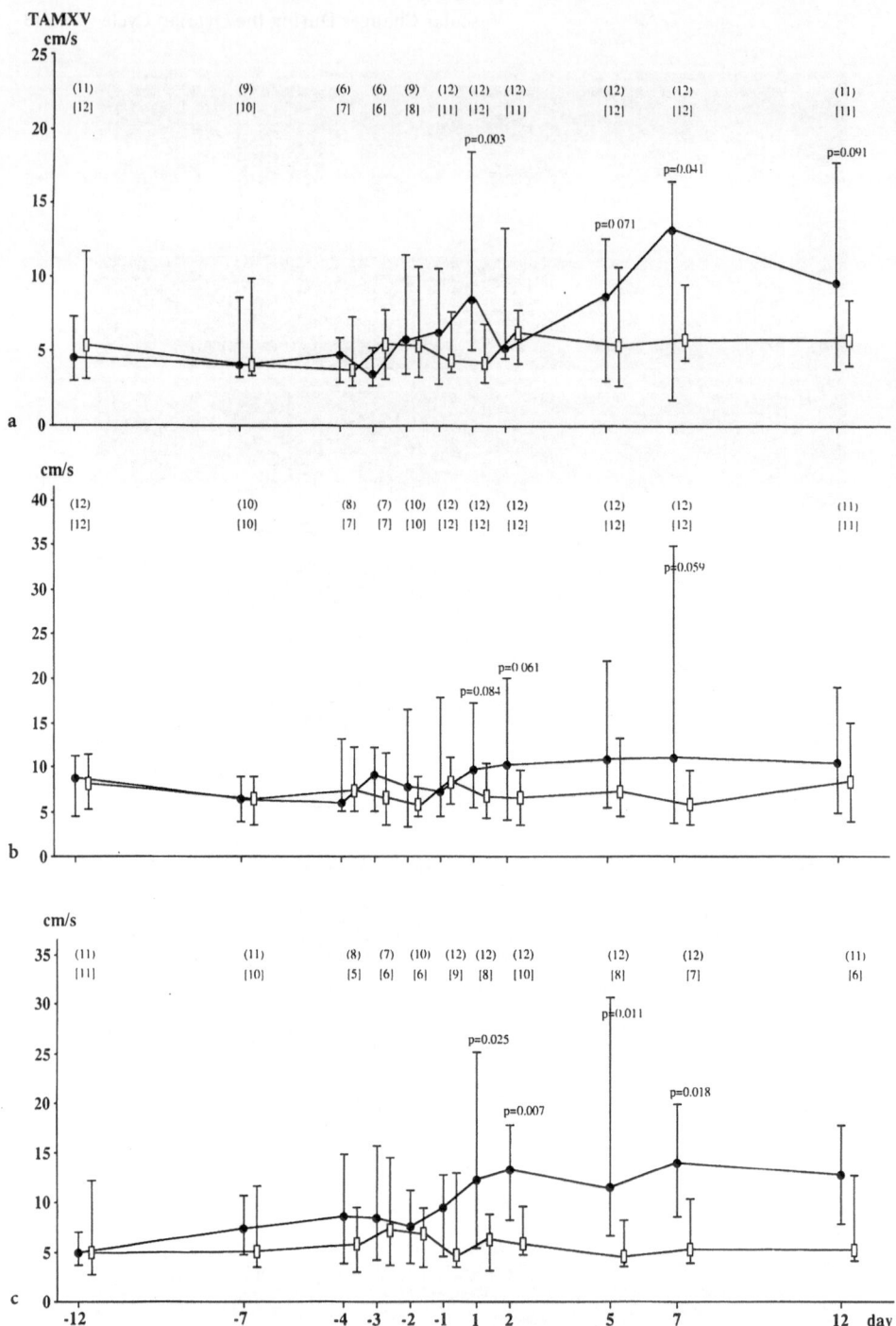

Fig. 4a–f. Time-averaged maximum velocity (*TAMXV*) and pulsatility index (*PI*) in the hilum (**a,d**), stroma (**b,e**) and wall of the largest follicle (**c,f**) of the dominant and non-dominant ovary. *Filled circles* represent the dominant and *open squares* the non-dominant ovary. Median, tenth and 90th percentile values are given. The figures in *brackets* denote the number of measurements in the dominant ovary, and the figures in *square brackets* the

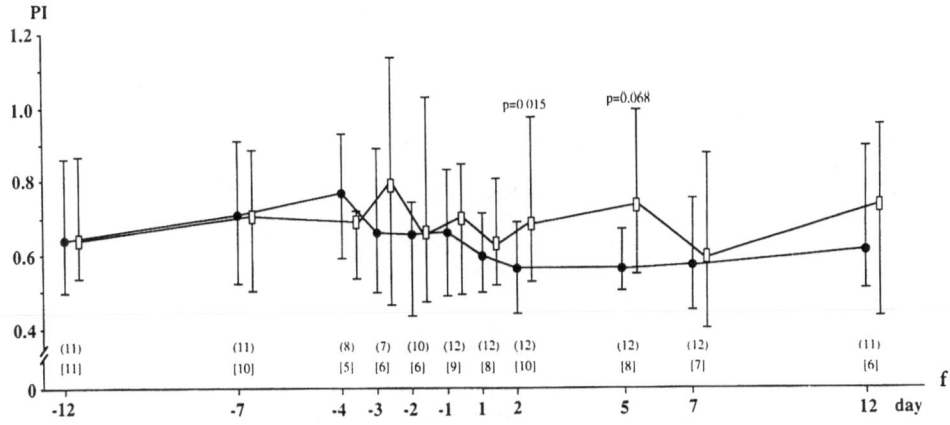

number of measurements in the non-dominant ovary. The results are expressed in relation to the time of presumed ovulation determined from the ultrasound image, the last day that the dominant follicle was visible on the ultrasound screen being day −1, and the first day that the corpus luteum was visible on the ultrasound screen day 1, etc. Ovulation was presumed to have occurred between the examinations on day −1 and day 1. (Slightly modified from [12]; published with permission from the Parthenon Publishing Company)

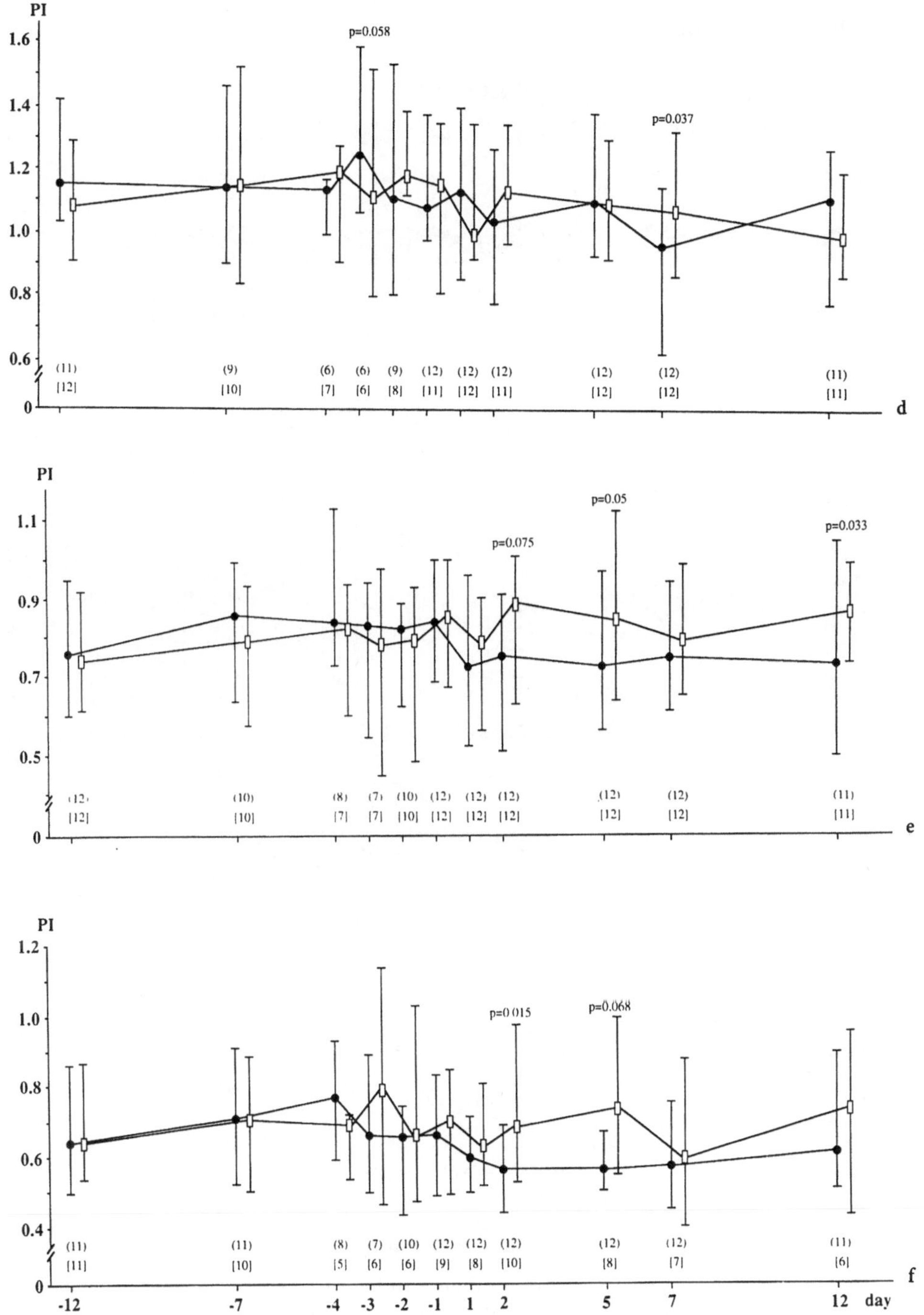

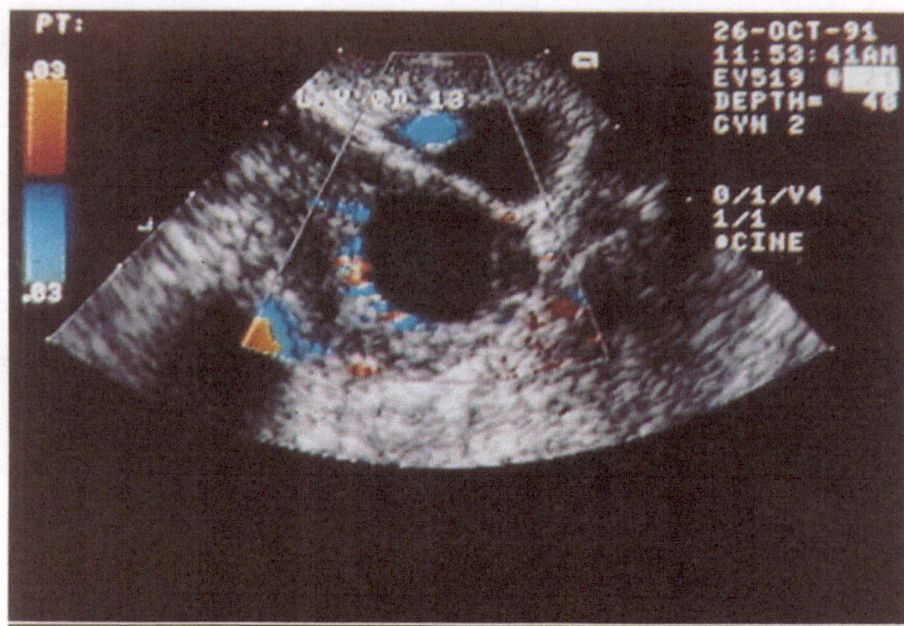

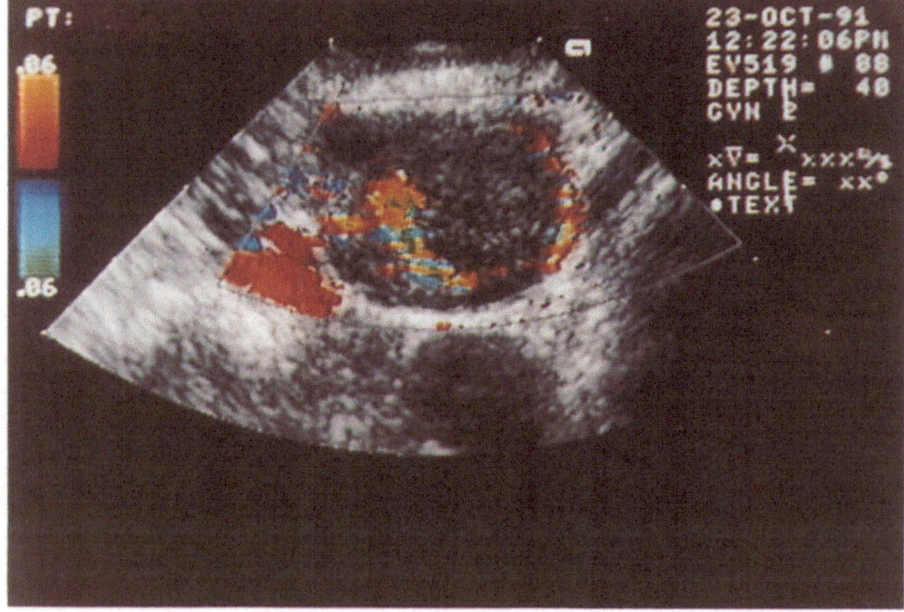

Fig. 5a,b. Colour Doppler images of the dominant follicle 4 days before follicular rupture (**a**) and of the corpus luteum 7 days after follicular rupture (**b**). Note the difference in thickness, length and intensity of the colour line outlining the wall of the dominant follicle and the corpus luteum. The equipment used was an Acuson 128 XP ultrasound system with a 5-MHz transvaginal probe. (From [12]; published with permission from the Parthenon Publishing Company)

have measured the true velocity of blood. However, we are confident that the changes and relative rather than absolute differences in velocity that we observed during the menstrual cycle reflected true changes in blood flow velocity. It is unlikely that the increased velocity of blood recorded in the dominant ovary and in the uterus in the luteal phase can have been due to our having inadvertently but consistently used a smaller insonation angle in the luteal than in the follicular phase. Thus, even though we cannot expect to measure true velocities of blood in small or tortuous vessels with the Doppler technique, useful qualitative evaluations of changes in velocity can almost certainly be made.

In conclusion, the results of published studies show that during the normal menstrual cycle dramatic changes occur in the blood circulation of the uterus and dominant ovary (as characterized by the colour Doppler image, the impedance index and the time-averaged maximum velocity or peak systolic velocity), whereas the blood circulation in the non-dominant ovary remains fairly constant. Knowledge of these circulatory changes in the uterus and adnexae during the normal menstrual cycle provides a basis for studies of pathological conditions in women of reproductive age (e.g. unexplained infertility, ovulation disturbances, polycystic ovary sydrome and adnexal tumours). However, given the many factors that may affect the results of Doppler measurements (e.g. the sampling technique and the sensitivity of the Doppler ultrasound system used), it would seem to be advisable for each laboratory to establish their own range of "normal values". This applies not only to values for blood flow velocity and impedance indices, but also to the evaluation of what constitutes a "normal" colour Doppler image of the uterus and ovaries.

References

1. Battaglia C, Larocca E, Lanzani A, Valentini M, Genazzani AR (1990) Doppler ultrasound studies of the uterine arteries in spontaneous and IVF stimulated ovarian cycles. Gynecol Endocrinol 4: 245–250
2. Bourne TH, Jurkovic D, Waterstone J, Campbell S, Collins WP (1991) Intrafollicular blood flow during human ovulation. Ultrasound Obstet Gynecol 1: 53–59
3. Collins W, Jurkovic D, Bourne T, Kurjak A, Campbell S (1991) Ovarian morphology, endocrine function and intra-follicular blood flow during the peri-ovulatory period. Hum Reprod 3: 319–324
4. Goswamy RK, Steptoe PC (1988) Doppler ultrasound studies of the uterine artery in spontaneous ovarian cycles. Hum Reprod 3: 721–726
5. Greisen G, Johansen, Ellison PH, Fredriksen PS, Mali J, Friis-Hansen B (1984) Cerebral blood flow in the newborn infant: comparison of Doppler ultrasound and 133 xenon clearance. J Pediatr 104: 411–418
6. Hansen NB, Stonestreet BS, Rosenkrantz TS, Oh W (1983) Validity of Doppler measurements of anterior cerebral artery blood flow velocity: correlation with brain blood flow in piglets. Pediatrics 72: 526–53
7. Hata K, Hata T, Senoh D, Makihara K, Aoki S, Takamiya O, Kitao M (1990) Change in ovarian arterial compliance during the human menstrual cycle assessed by Doppler ultrasound. Br J Obstet Gynaecol 97: 163–166
8. Kremkau FW (1990) Doppler ultrasound. Principles and instruments. Saunders, Philadelphia, pp 113–114, 138

9. Mercé LT, Garcés D, Barco MJ, de la Fuente F (1992) Intraovarian Doppler velocimetry in ovulatory, dysovulatory and anovulatory cycles. Ultrasound Obstet Gynecol 2: 197–202
10. Rosenberg AA, Narayanan V, Jones MD (1985) Comparison of anterior cerebral artery blood flow velocity and cerebral blood flow during hypoxia. Pediatr Res 19: 67–70
11. Scholtes MCW, Wladimiroff JW, van Rijen HJM, Hop WCJ (1989) Uterine and ovarian flow velocity waveforms in the normal menstrual cycle: a transvaginal study. Fertil Steril 52: 981–985
12. Sladkevicius P, Valentin L, Marsàl K (1993) Blood flow velocity in uterine and ovarian arteries during the normal menstrual cycle. Ultrasound Obstet Gynecol 3: 199–208
13. Steer CV, Campbell S, Pampiglione JS, Kingsland CR, Mason BA, Collins WP (1990) Transvaginal colour flow imaging of the uterine arteries during the ovarian and menstrual cycles. Hum Reprod 5: 391–395
14. Taylor KJW, Burns PN, Wells PNT, Conway DI, Hull MGR (1985) Ultrasound Doppler flow studies of the ovarian and uterine arteries. Br J Obstet Gynaecol 92: 240–246

Ovulation and the Periovulatory Follicle

T.H. Bourne, S. Athanasiou, and B. Bauer

Introduction

The introduction and use of transvaginal colour flow imaging has facilitated the study of vascular changes within the pelvis. The follicle and corpus luteum of the ovary and the endometrium of the uterus are the only areas in a normal adult body where angiogenesis (the development of new blood vessels) occurs to any significant extent; the same process occurs during the growth of carcinomas. The ability to recognise these early vascular changes with colour Doppler is facilitating the diagnosis of pelvic cancers as well as normal and abnormal ovarian and uterine function. It seems likely that this technique will lead to a greater understanding of how vessel growth is involved in reproductive pathophysiology. The ability to monitor changes in vascularity may enable the development of methods to inhibit or enhance angiogenic activity in vivo.

This chapter will attempt to briefly outline the principles of transvaginal colour Doppler and its practical use, before discussing its applications regarding the study of vascular changes around the time of presumed ovulation.

Technique

For some time research efforts have been directed towards developing techniques to observe vascular changes within the human pelvis. This work has been centred on the use of Doppler ultrasound, the principles and physics of which have been reviewed [25]. Whilst B-mode imaging has progressed to allow structures to be inspected in "real time", up to now the use of pulsed or spectral Doppler has required a considerable length of time to select the point that best represents the vessel or area of tissue being investigated. The operator is limited by the fact that flow information is narrowed to the highly restricted pulsed Doppler range gate from which the blood flow data are obtained, and as a result sampling errors are not uncommon. These limitations have made the study of small vessels and minor vascular changes very difficult to carry out in a reproducible fashion. This is of particular relevance to performing reproducible studies of ovarian function. Colour Doppler solves many of these problems. The B-mode image is divided into many pixels, and the Doppler flow parameters for each of the pixels on the screen are demonstrated in "real time". The Doppler information is colour frequency coded, and a colour converter assigns colour based on the direction and variance of the detected frequency shifts. Red usually indicates flow towards the transducer, and blue away. The brightness of the colour is proportional to the velocity of flow within the vessel, whilst turbulent flow may appear as various shades of green [18]. In this way regions of vascularisation can be located anatomically as areas of colour and a pulsed Doppler range gate then placed over the area of interest to provide flow velocity waveforms for conventional analysis.

There is a tendency towards overenthusiasm regarding the applications of colour Doppler. Whilst it is an elegant way of displaying Doppler information, at the present time it is not possible to quantify colour Doppler. It must be remembered that it acts to identify vessels such that a sample volume gate can be used to obtain flow velocity waveforms. We therefore rely for data collection on the analysis of these frequency spectra. The conventional indices of resistance index (RI) and the pulsatility index (PI) are both thought to reflect changes in impedance to flow distal to the point of sampling [23, 24]. In many cases these indices fail to show any differences when comparing physiological and pathological processes. In a study by Bower et al. in 1993 [6], the presence or absence of a notch in the uterine artery waveform was far more predictive of future pregnancy outcome than the use of either the RI or PI. Subtle differences in waveform shape and character are lost in the spectrum analysis. It is probable that this is useful information; new ways to analyze this Doppler information are needed.

The safety aspects of transvaginal colour Doppler must not be forgotten. In general the power output of colour Doppler units is not a cause for concern, and for most units the spacial peak average intensity (SPTA) is of the order of 30 mW/cm^2. This is well within the highest limit recommended by the Food and Drug Administration (FDA) for use in obstetrics. There are, however, concerns regarding the use of transvaginal pulsed Doppler units, and a number of machines currently available have power outputs above the FDA guidelines when used at high power settings. Such power outputs are not required to obtain good waveforms using vaginal Doppler, and the power should be reduced to the lowest level possible. The trend towards the display of power output levels on screen is to be recommended. The use of transvaginal colour Doppler should, if anything, lead to safety advantages. By reducing the time required to find and sample a vessel, the total exposure of the area of interest to ultrasound should be reduced. Such a discussion of safety is not just of academic interest, as little is known about the effects of Doppler ultrasound on the ovary. In the absence of any proof of safety, exposure of the ovary to pulsed Doppler ultrasound should be kept to the minimum required to gain the information necessary for any study.

Practical Application

Often the identification of small subtle vascular points within the ovary using colour Doppler is made difficult by movement artefact. The proximity of the ovaries to the highly pulsatile iliac vessels makes this inevitable, although with experience it is possible to discriminate between areas of "true" colour that represent blood flow and artefact. It is important to remember that any data obtained using transvaginal colour Doppler is of little value if the vessel sampled has been incorrectly identified. There are certainly published data claiming to relate to ovarian artery flow, when the waveforms shown are clearly iliac in origin. All of the major pelvic vessels have characteristic waveform "signatures" [22], and it is easy to become familiar with these by placing a continuous wave Doppler probe on the vessels in question at the time of laparotomy (Fig. 1). It is our experience that it is extremely difficult to measure blood flow in the ovarian artery; it is not clear whether this is because the angle of insonation is suboptimal or because the blood flow velocity is very low, or a combination of both. Most ovarian blood flow data refer to areas of intra-ovarian vascularity rather than the ovarian artery itself. When interrogating such areas of vascularity, the brightest point of colour must be sampled to obtain the highest velocity flows. The probe can then be angled very slightly to maximise the amplitude of the waveform. It is important not to accept the first measurable waveform as representative of blood flow within the tissue being studied, and it is worth spending a little time to ensure that the vascular area with the highest velocity and lowest impedance has been sampled. In this way highly reproducible measurements of the RI, PI and velocity can be made. The issue of velocity measurements is an important one. In the presence of angiogenesis it is clear that the angle of insonation of these small vessels will not be known; however, it now generally accepted that enough of these small vessels will be approached from a low or zero angle to allow reproducible maximum systolic velocity measurements to be made.

The interrelated effects of vascularisation are illustrated in Fig. 2. It is clear that the growth of new vessels or the development of existing ones forms a common thread throughout many areas of reproductive pathophysiology. It is clear just by observing biological events such as angiogenesis and apoptosis that such events are common to both physiological and pathological changes in the ovary. It is thus important to understand these normal events before turning our attention exclusively to the situation in the presence of pathology.

The Ovary Around the Time of Ovulation

Some of the potential applications of transvaginal colour Doppler in infertility have been discussed [9]. At the present time there are no useful morphological markers of impending ovulation, although ultrasound has been used to monitor follicular growth and rupture as well as observe the formation of the early corpus luteum [19]. Other workers have suggested that details of corpus luteum morphology can be used to identify those associated with plasma progesterone concentrations of 35 nmol/l or more [17], although there are no data to indicate whether these same criteria would select those corpora lutea likely to respond normally to signals from a developing trophoblast or embryo. Whilst the ability to detect that a follicle has ruptured is being used to develop practical self-tests for

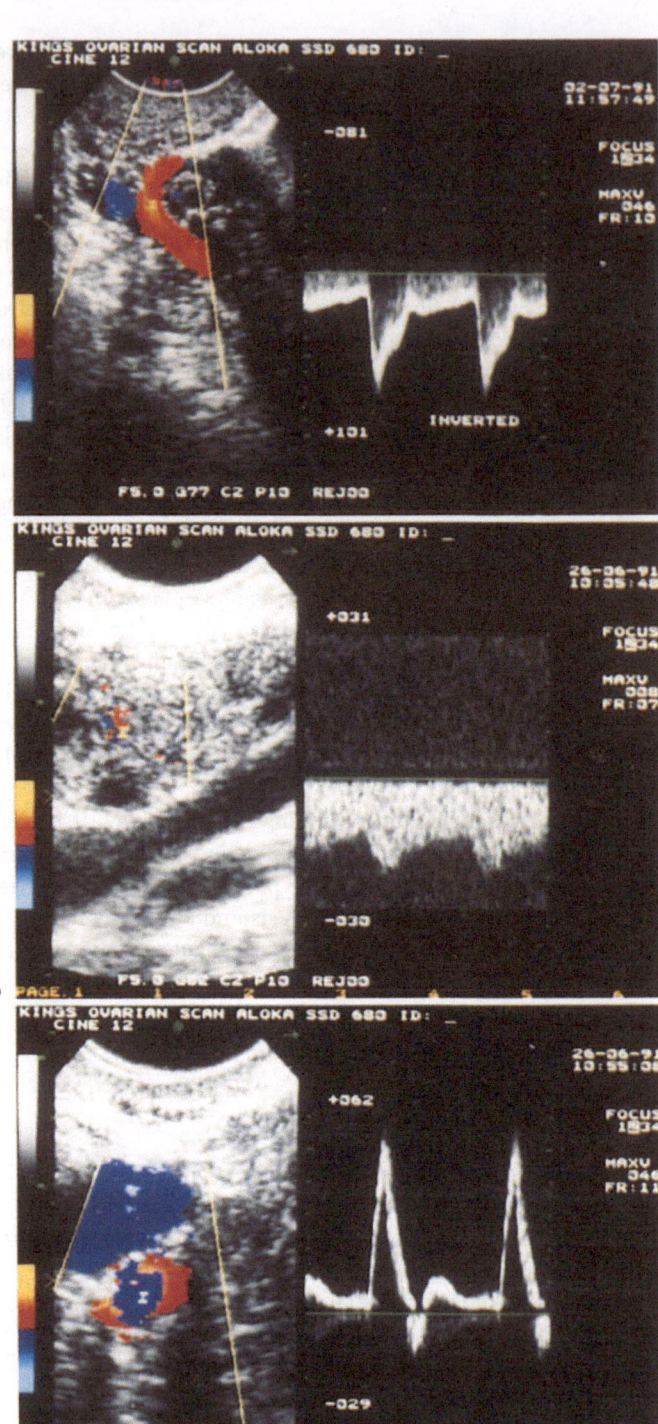

Fig. 1a–c. Typical "signature" flow velocity waveforms from the internal iliac artery (**c**), the uterine artery (**a**), and from within a solid corpus luteum (**b**). Note that the pulsed Doppler range gate is positioned within the stroma of the ovary

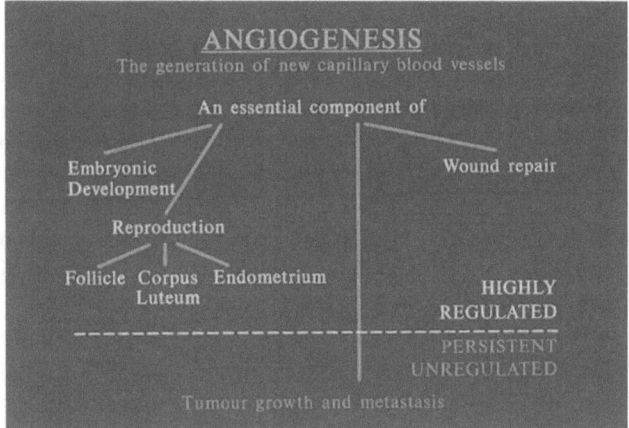

Fig. 2. The related effects of angiogenesis in reproductive pathophysiology. It is possible that a greater understanding of what regulates normal "physiological" angiogenesis will also have implications for the diagnosis and treatment of pathological processes. Transvaginal colour Doppler offers a relatively non-invasive way of monitoring these processes

potential fertility, there is still a need for a technique that can predict (and possibly detect) the release or possible retention of a viable oocyte at the time of follicular rupture. Transvaginal colour Doppler has been used to monitor sequential changes in intrafollicular blood flow in the periovulatory period, and the data obtained related to defined biochemical indices. It is hoped that it will be possible to use information about ovarian blood flow both to predict ovulation and to investigate ovulatory dysfunction.

Previous studies have shown that it is possible to assess ovarian blood flow during the normal menstrual cycle [11]. The study by Hata et al. using transabdominal pulsed Doppler showed significant changes in ovarian blood flow in the ovarian cycle; in particular, there was a marked drop in blood flow impedance within the ovary during the late follicular and luteal phase of the cycle. Although these authors interpret their data as being from the ovarian artery, it is more likely that serial measurements of intra-ovarian flow have been recorded. Using transvaginal colour Doppler, these areas of vascularity can be clearly visualised on the follicle rim or within or around the corpus luteum. Transvaginal pulsed Doppler has been subsequently used to record blood flow in the corpus luteum in in vitro fertilisation (IVF) patients following embryo transfer [2]. In the absence of colour flow imaging the authors had to move the sample volume gate (of 3.5 mm) over the ovarian stroma until suitable waveforms had been obtained. Again, the waveforms are therefore more likely to reflect intra-ovarian rather than ovarian artery blood flow. Impedance to blood flow was measured on days 3 and 10 following embryo transfer, and significantly higher impedance to flow observed in the corpora lutea of women who failed to become pregnant.

Transvaginal colour Doppler has since been used to intensively monitor vascular events in the periovulatory follicle [8]. Colour Doppler facilitates the detection of small vascular areas in the ovarian stroma and follicle rim that are easy to miss when applying a pulsed Doppler range gate "blind" (Fig. 3). In this study the aim was to assess each patient every 3–4 h from the time of the serum luteinizing hormone (LH) surge up to the formation of the corpus luteum. Blood flow velocity waveforms from the follicular rim were first seen at the time of the LH surge (or oestradiol [E_2] peak). We were able to demonstrate the sequential increase in vascularity in the follicle rim from the time of the LH rise, at its peak and finally just prior to ovulation and the formation of the corpus luteum. These observations represent the first report of the changes in intrafollicular vascularity over the periovulatory period in the human female. Subsequent work confirmed and extended these preliminary data. Ten women with apparently normal ovarian cycles were studied [7]. The time intervals between the mean values for the peak systolic velocity and serum LH and progesterone (P) relative to the mean time of follicular rupture are shown in Fig. 4. There is a tendency for intrafollicular blood velocity to increase approximately 29 h before the time of follicular rupture. This rise continues for at least 72 h after the formation of the corpus haemorrhagicum and is reflected in the colour Doppler information obtained at this time (Fig. 5). The mean changes in peak systolic velocity appear to follow the mean rise in circulatory LH by approximately 12 h. These data are supported by other workers [14]. In this study of both stimulated and spontaneous ovarian cycles, peak systolic blood velocity within the ovary also tended to increase on the day of ovulation. It is of interest that this group observed a significant decrease in impedance to flow within the ovary at the time of formation of the corpus luteum; there were no differences in blood flow indices between spontaneous and stimulated cycles. Sladkevicius

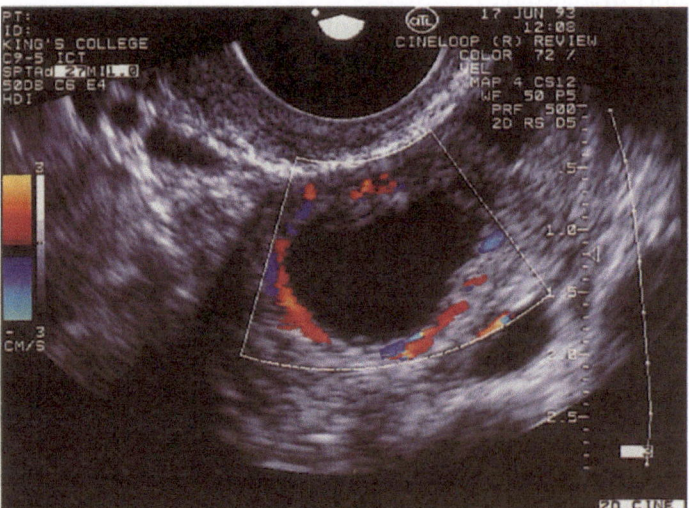

Fig. 3. Intense vascularity around the periphery of a follicle just prior to ovulation. The area of maximum velocity is located at 5 o'clock on the follicle wall. The colour at this point is brighter and just turning to green and yellow

et al. [20] also found an increase in peak systolic blood velocity in the follicle wall the day before presumed ovulation, with little change in the pulsatility index. This paper is discussed in more detail in the chapter by Valentin. These results are given credence by studies of ovarian blood flow and volume in laboratory animals [21] and the fact that red blood cells have been seen in the granulosa cell layer between the time of the LH peak and presumed ovulation [3].

A report of the vascular changes at the time of ovulation shows increased vascularity on the inner most rim of the follicle (Fig. 3) and a coincident surge in blood flow velocity just prior to follicular rupture [4]. This may represent the dilatation of new vessels that have developed between the relatively vascular theca cell layer and the normally hypoxic granulosa cell layer of the follicle. It is of interest that these marked differences in peak systolic velocity occurred in the presence of a relatively constant PI. This supports the view that peak systolic velocity is the most accurate reflection of vascular events within the ovary. It seems unlikely that such rapid changes in systolic velocity represent actual

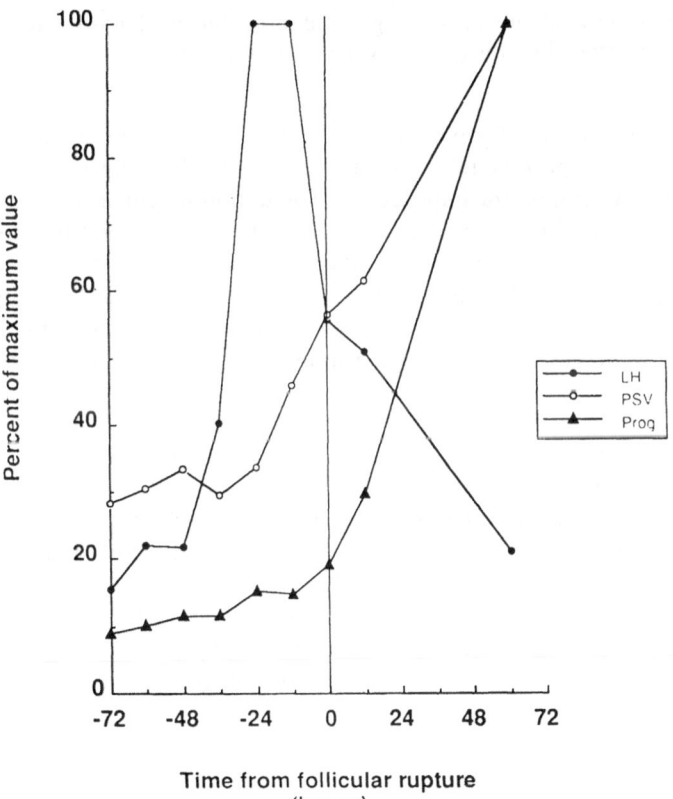

Fig. 4. The pattern of changes in peak systolic velocity (*PSV*; within the follicle) and peripheral serum luteinising hormone (*LH*) and progesterone (*P*), relative to the mean time for follicular rupture (from [7] with the permission of the American Fertility Society)

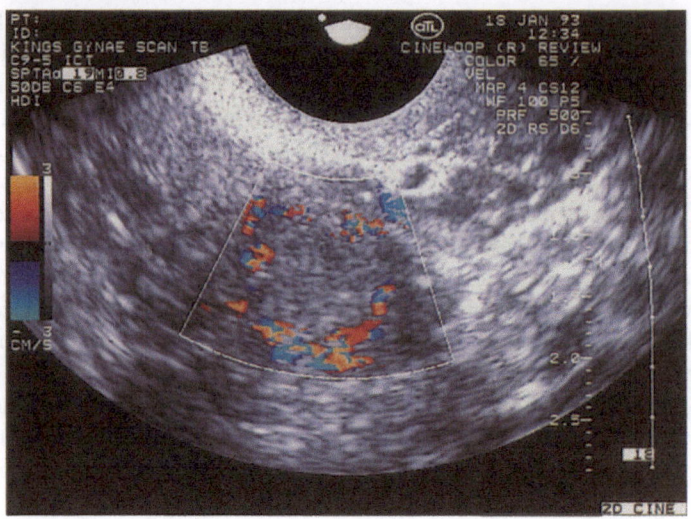

Fig. 5. An ordered ring of vascularity surrounding a solid corpus luteum. It is of interest to contrast this with the irregular branching vessels demonstrated in early ovarian cancer

neoangiogenesis itself, but more probably an alteration in the tone of existing vascular beds. The rise in peak systolic velocity was variable but universal. This novel finding may have important implications. Disruption or enhancement of these vascular changes would have profound effects on the oxygen concentration across the follicular epithelium [10] with significant consequences for cell function. It was clear at this time that more studies would be needed to determine whether these changes in peak systolic blood velocity around the time of the E_2 peak and LH rise are necessary for follicular rupture and the release of a viable oocyte.

During our studies we also noted that there was a period after follicular rupture when the flow velocity waveforms became more ill-defined or "fuzzy". It had been reported that this effect could be used to differentiate between ovulatory and non-ovulatory cycles, a proposition that has yet to be substantiated [16]. Other workers [15] have studied earlier events in the ovarian cycle and reported that the leading follicle has evidence of increased blood flow relative to other follicles well before the LH peak. This is consistent with the view that neovascularisation occurs relatively early in the ovarian cycle and that the dramatic changes in vascularity are a reflection of the local action of vasoactive factors on this pre-existing vascular bed.

Ovulatory Dysfunction

We have reported one case of drug-associated luteinized unruptured follicle (LUF), and these preliminary data suggested reduction in vascularisation and a

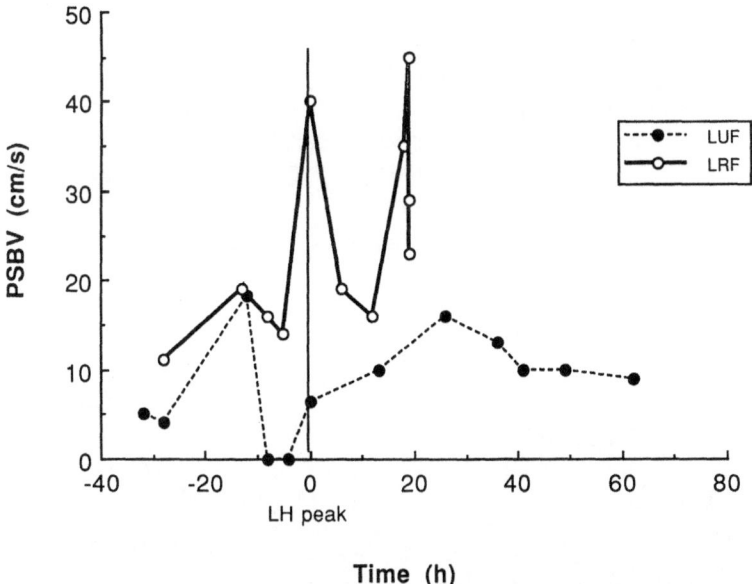

Fig. 6. Changes in peak systolic blood velocity (*PSBV*) within a luteinised ruptured follicle (*LRF*) and an luteinised unruptured follicle (*LUF*) associated with the ingestion of paracetamol (from Fig. 4 of [5], with permission from of the International Society for Ultrasound in Obstetrics and Gynecology)

failure of the blood flow velocity to peak in the immediate preovulatory period [5] (Fig. 6). We felt that this might be consistent with the view that the changes in oxygen tension within the follicle brought about by angiogenesis are necessary for normal ovulation to occur. Accordingly, we have since studied a further eight women [1]. The same protocol was used, except that once the leading follicle had reached 18 mm, indomethacin (50 mg tds) or paracetamol (500 mg qds) was given for a period of 72 h. Indomethacin was given on the basis of previous reports associating its use with the formation of luteinized unruptured follicles [13]. It is of interest that all (*n* = 4) of the women receiving indomethacin developed LUF, but did not demonstrate any reduction in peak systolic velocity to the follicle. Furthermore, oocytes subsequently removed from these follicles were of high quality. In contrast, those taking paracetamol (*n* = 4) ovulated with just one exception and displayed a significant reduction in peak systolic velocity to the follicle. In the one case where it was possible to retrieve an oocyte from this group, it was necrotic. It is clear that we were premature in our hypothesis that a change in peak systolic blood velocity is necessary for normal follicular rupture to take place. It now seems to us more likely that this alteration in vasculature is in some way necessary for the normal development of the oocyte. Our preliminary data observing the peak systolic blood velocity in individual follicles of stimulated ovaries gives anecdotal support for this view (Nargund and Bourne, unpublished data). Of 72 follicles

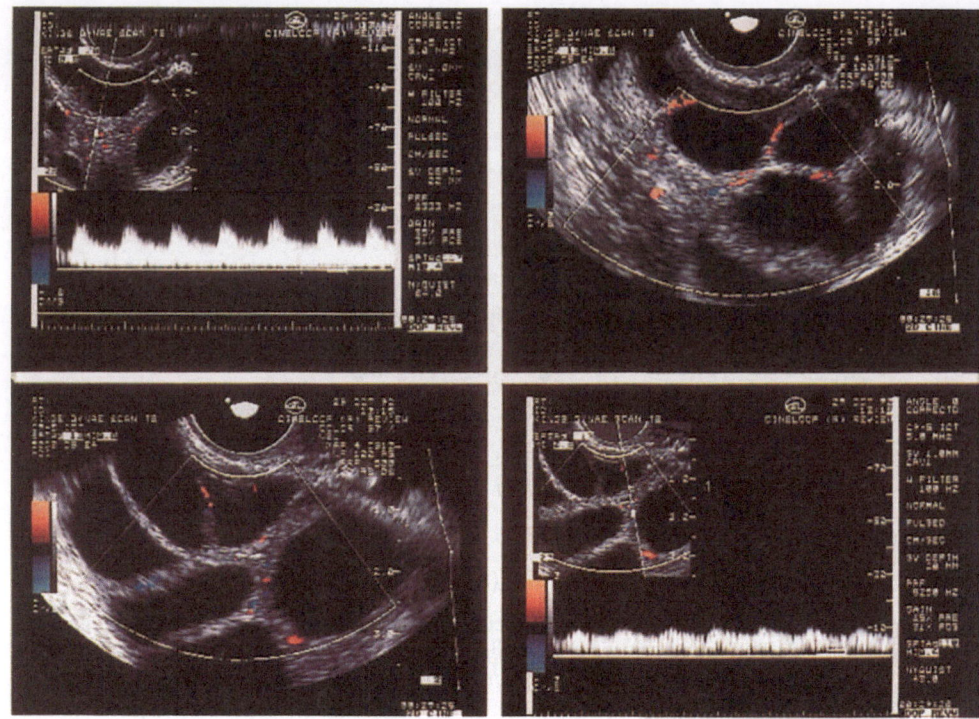

Fig. 7. Colour Doppler images showing vascularity within a stimulated ovary. Note that pulsed Doppler has generated waveforms of variable velocity from near different follicles

studied, there is a clear correlation between the peak systolic blood velocity in the follicle and the quality of the subsequent oocyte that is obtained at egg collection Fig. 7. These findings are preliminary. However, it is tempting to speculate that if we can manipulate ovarian blood flow at critical times of the cycle, it may be possible to alter oocyte development with the aim of either enhancing or diminishing the possibility of pregnancy occurring.

Conclusions

Transvaginal colour Doppler may be used to monitor hormonal and other methods of increasing or decreasing intrafollicular blood flow. Steroids that inhibit angiogenesis in the presence of heparin have already been described [12], and if the process of ovulation could be inhibited independently of the main pathways of steroidogenesis then novel methods of contraception might be envisaged. When the cellular and molecular mechanisms of neoangiogenesis in healthy and pathological tissues have been elucidated it will be possible to influence these processes to advantage. Initial evidence suggests that transvaginal colour flow mapping may be used to monitor progress towards these objectives. It is further hoped that transvaginal colour Doppler will facilitate the study of other aspects of ovarian function such as follicular recruitment and corpus luteum development and failure.

It is clear that changes in tissue vascularity are fundamental to many aspects of normal ovarian function. The preliminary data with transvaginal colour Doppler suggests that it may provide a relatively non-invasive tool for their detailed study. Prospective data are now needed to assess whether ways can be found to alter these vascular processes either to enhance or reduce the chances of a couple achieving a pregnancy.

Acknowledgements. We are grateful to Keymed Ltd. (Southend, UK) and to the ALOKA Co. Ltd. (Tokyo, Japan) for the use of their ultrasound equipment. We would like to thank Zeneca Ltd. and Schering Health Care for their support of the gynaecological ultrasound clinic.

References

1. Athanasiou S, Bourne TH, Khalid A, Hagström HG, Okokon EV, Crayford TJB, Campbell S, Collins WP (1995) Effects of indomethacin on follicular structure and function over the peri-ovulatory period. Fertil Steril (in press)
2. Baber RJ, McSweeney MB, Gill RW, Porter RN, Picker RH, Warren PS, Kossoff G, Saunders DM (1988) Transvaginal pulsed Doppler ultrasound assessment of blood flow to the corpus luteum in IVF patients following embryo transfer. Br J Obstet Gynaecol 95: 1226–1230
3. Bomsel-Helmreich O, Gougeon A, Thebault A, Salarelli D, Milgrom E, Frydman R, Papiernik E (1979) Healthy and atretic human follicles in the preovulatory phase: differences in evolution of follicular morphology and steroid content of follicular fluid. J Clin Endocrinol Metab 48: 686–694
4. Bourne TH, Jurkovic D, Waterstone J, Campbell S, Collins WP (1991) Intrafollicular blood flow during human ovulation. Ultrasound Obstet Gynecol 1: 53–59
5. Bourne TH, Reynolds K, Jurkovic D, Waterstone J, Campbell S, Collins WP (1991) Paracetamol-associated luteinised unruptured follicle syndrome: effect on intra-follicular blood flow. Ultrasound Obstet Gynecol 1: 420–425
6. Bower S, Schuchter K, Vyas S, Campbell S (1993) The study of uterine artery blood flow to predict IUGR and pregnancy induced hypertension. Obstet Gynecol 82: 78–83
7. Campbell S, Bourne TH, Waterstone J, Reynolds K, Crayford TJB, Jurkovic D, Okokon EV, Collins WP (1993) Transvaginal color blood flow imaging of the periovulatory follicle. Fertil Steril 60: 433–438
8. Collins W, Jurkovic D, Bourne TH, Kurjak A, Campbell S (1991) Ovarian morphology, endocrine function and intra-follicular blood flow during the peri-ovulatory period. Hum Reprod 6: 319–324
9. Fleischer AC (1991) Ultrasound imaging 2000: assessment of utero-ovarian blood flow with transvaginal color Doppler sonography; potential clinical applications in infertility. Fertil Steril 55: 684–691
10. Gosden RG, Byatt-Smith JG (1986) Oxygen concentration across the ovarian follicular epithelium: model, predictions and implications. Hum Reprod 1: 65–68
11. Hata K, Hata T, Senoh D, Makihara K, Aoki S, Takamiya O, Kitao A (1990) Change in ovarian arterial compliance during the human menstrual cycle by Doppler ultrasound. Br J Obstet Gynaecol 97: 163–166

12. Ingber DE, Madri JA, Folkman J (1986) A possible mechanism for inhibition of angiogenesis by angiostatic steroids: induction of capillary basement membrane dissolution. Endocrinology 119: 1768-1775
13. Killick S, Elstein M (1987) Pharmacologic production of luteinised unruptured follicle by prostaglandin synthetase inhibitors. Fertil Steril 47: 773-777
14. Kupesic S, Kurjak A (1993) Uterine and ovarian perfusion during the periovulatory period assessed by transvaginal color Doppler. Fertil Steril 60: 439-443
15. Kurjak A, Kupesic S, Schulman H, Zalud I (1991) Transvaginal color flow Doppler in the assessment of ovarian and uterine blood flow in infertile women. Fertil Steril 56: 870-873
16. Merce LT, Garces D, Barco MJ, de la Fuente F (1992) Intraovarian Doppler velocimetry, dysovulatory and anovulatory cycles. Ultrasound Obstets Gynecol 2: 197-202
17. Nakata M, Selstam G, Olufsson J, Backstrom T (1992) Investigation of the human corpus luteum by ultrasonography - a proposed scheme for clinical investigation. Ultrasound Obstet Gynecol 2: 190-196
18. Omoto R, Kasai C (1987) Physics and instrumentation of Doppler colour flow mapping. Echocardiogr Rev Cardiovasc Ultrasound 4: 467-483
19. Queenan JT, O'Brian GD, Bains LM, Simpson J, Collins WP, Campbell S (1980) Ultrasound scanning of ovaries to detect ovulation in women. Fertil Steril 34: 99-105
20. Sladkevicius P, Valentin L, Marsal K (1993) Blood flow velocity in the uterine and ovarian arteries during the menstrual cycle. Ultrasound Obstet Gynecol 3: 199-208
21. Tanaka N, Espey LL, Okamura H (1989) Increase in ovarian blood volume during ovulation in the gonadotrophin-primed immature rat. Biol Reprod 40: 762-768
22. Taylor KJW, Burns PN, Wells PNT, Conway DI, Hull MGR (1985) Ultrasound Doppler flow studies of the ovarian and uterine arteries. Br J Obstet Gynaecol 92: 240-246
23. Thompson RS, Trudinger BJ, Cook CM (1988) Doppler ultrasound waveform indices: A/B ratio, pulsatility index and Pourcelot ratio. Br J Obstet Gynaecol 95: 581-588
24. Trudinger BJ, Thompson RS (1991) Do velocity indices measure resistance? Ultrasound Obstets Gynecol 3: 160-161
25. Wells PNT (1989) Doppler ultrasound in medical diagnosis. Br J Radiology 62: 399-420

The Study of Ovarian Tumours

T.H. Bourne, K. Gruböck, and A. Tailor

Introduction

The use of transvaginal colour Doppler to characterise ovarian masses has perhaps attracted more attention that any other of its applications. Certainly the introduction of a technique that would reliably discriminate between benign and malignant tumours would be of benefit. The routine use of transvaginal ultrasonography has presented gynaecologists with the difficult problem of managing asymptomatic ovarian cysts found by such opportunistic examinations. Ultrasound-based ovarian cancer screening programmes have similar potential difficulties. For symptomatic masses, important management decisions are now being made according to their ultrasound appearances. Observation, ultrasound-guided cyst puncture, laparoscopic surgery or formal laparotomy are four of the options available for clinicians treating an ovarian cyst. The patient's age, the presence or absence of a family history of cancer, tumour marker expression and B-mode ultrasound appearance as well as the size of any lesion are all of importance. Yet at any international ultrasound meeting there are lectures stating that information derived from transvaginal colour Doppler ultrasonography is all that is needed to make clinical decisions about these patients. Is this optimism justified? Furthermore, does transvaginal colour Doppler provide us with a better indication of the nature of an ovarian cyst than other approaches to the problem? This chapter will try to address these issues.

Discriminating Benign from Malignant Masses

Preliminary Work

Changes in tissue vascularity, mediated by angiogenic factors, are associated with the early stages of ovarian oncogenesis. Recent studies with transgenic mice have shown that for at least one type of cancer, angiogenesis occurs during the transition from hyperplasia to neoplasia [15]. An inhibitor of angiogenesis has also been found that is produced by cells when they are capable of expressing an active cancer-suppressing gene [27]. This evidence suggests that angiogenesis may well be an obligate event in the earliest stages of ovarian carcinoma. More recently a strong correlation has been observed between the malignant nature of a series of ovarian tumours and the expression of messenger RNA for platelet-derived end-othelial growth factor (thymidine phosphorylase) [28]. In animal models, Doppler techniques have been used to identify areas of altered vascularisation within tumours as small as 50 mg [26]. In this study, vascular morphology was further evaluated by digital angiography; this technique demonstrated coincidence be-tween the site of high-velocity, low-impedance signals and the presence of arterio-venous anastomoses [29]. Preliminary data suggests that it may be possible to detect the vascular changes associated with early ovarian cancers using transvaginal colour Doppler. In malignant lesions, blood flow can be demon-strated throughout diastole, probably reflecting a decrease in impedance to flow distal to the point of sampling. A possible explanation for this is that the new vessels associated with carcinoma have limited vascular tone due to the absence of the tunica media, and as a result they form low-impedance shunts. On the basis of this work it was hoped that it would be possible to characterise benign and malig-nant lesions on the basis of their vascularity.

To investigate this possibility, Bourne et al. [1] studied 30 women with no apparent pelvic pathology and 18 women with ovarian tumours. All cases of invasive cancer showed evidence of neovascularisation with low-impedance blood flow. One serous cystadenoma of borderline malignancy did not demonstrate an abnormal blood flow pattern, and there was one false-positive test result (a benign teratoma). Two of the invasive cancers were at stage Ia, suggesting that this tech-nique can detect ovarian cancer when it is still confined to the capsule of the ovary. These results were supported by the work of Kurjak et al. [19], who studied infertile women with presumed normal pelvic anatomy and patients with known pelvic masses. Low-impedance intra-tumoural blood flow was seen in four cases of unstaged primary ovarian cancer; the resistance index (RI) was used as an index of impedance to flow and was below 0.40 in all cases. There was one false-positive test result (a granulosa cell tumour) amongst the 15 benign cystic lesions that were studied. The authors regard an RI value of 0.40 as a significant cut-off, values below this being thought to have a high predictive value for carcinoma.

Cut-off Values for Indices of Impedance

The data of Hata et al. [17] suggest that the appropriate cut-off values to deter-mine normal and abnormal blood flow within the ovary have yet to be determined. In eight cases of ovarian cancer, the mean RI value was 0.503 ± 0.216. It is of interest that this group was unable to discriminate between the blood flow of a corpus luteum cyst, an endometrioid ovarian cyst and carcinoma. The same au-thors point out that in one case, internal iliac blood flow was mistaken for blood flow within the ovary, a common and important source of error. Data from our own clinic (Table 1) also demonstrate a clear overlap between the blood flow within normal physiological ovarian cystic lesions and carcinoma [12]. The use of an arbitrary cut-off value of 0.40 seems likely to result in a number of both false-positive and -negative results. Kurjak and Zalud [20] have also presented data on

Table 1. The resistance index (RI), pulsatility index (PI), and peak systolic velocity of preovulatory follicles, corpora lutea and early ovarian carcinomas

	Follicle (post LH) n = 12		Corpora lutea n = 30		Early ovarian cancer n = 7	
Variable	Mean	Range	Mean	Range	Mean	Range
Resistance index (RI)	0.48	0.36–0.58	0.43	0.28–0.54	0.46	0.33–0.78
Pulsatility index (PI)	0.62	0.39–0.99	0.56	0.30–0.73	0.61	0.40–0.96
Peak systolic velocity (cm/s)	26.1	14.3–45.2	43.2	16.1–73.4	44.0	35.6–57.5*

*$n = 3$.

the colour Doppler findings in 624 benign and 56 malignant ovarian masses. Presumed neovascularisation was demonstrated in six out of seven stage I primary ovarian cancers, and in 48 of 49 of the other malignant lesions in the study. In all of the cases where neovascularisation was seen, the RI value was again less than 0.40. In another series of seven cases of stage I ovarian carcinomas, neovascularisation was seen in all invasive carcinomas; the details of each case as well as their RI values are seen in Table 2 [2]. From these data it can be seen that using a cut-off value of 0.40 would have led to a number of false-negative diagnoses of cancer. In this context, the work of Tekay and Joupilla [30] is of some interest. Their data suggest that the use of arbitrary discriminatory cut-off values of RI and pulsatility index (PI) do not discriminate between benign and malignant tumours. According to these results classifying an ovarian tumour on the basis of an RI value of less than 0.4 would detect less than 40% of malignancies. It is difficult to explain the huge discrepancies between studies, especially when the data of Tekay and Joupilla are contrasted with a further study by Kurjak et al. [21] of 14 317 symptomatic and asymptomatic women. Of the 8620 asymptomatic women recruited to this study, 7495 were premenopausal. Yet only one false-positive test result and two false-negative test results were recorded. This is an extraordinary overall test performance. No other group has been able to replicate these data.

Other Ultrasound Criteria to Characterise Masses

Certainly one criticism of colour Doppler is that the operator is never blind to the B-mode image. There is a tendency to search harder for low-impedance vessels from a lesion with a "malignant" appearance than a "benign-looking" simple unilocular cyst. Other workers [14] have associated the presence or absence of a notch in the flow velocity waveform from the ovary with the likelihood of malignancy. This approach also has limitations. If a flow velocity waveform is obtained from a simple unilocular (and so probably benign) cyst, it will come from around

Table 2. Early stage ovarian cancers examined by transvaginal colour Doppler showing intraovarian indices of impedance to blood flow

Case no	Age	Menopausal status	Histological classification	FIGO stage	RI	PI	PSV
1	63	post	Borderline serous cystadenocarcinoma	Ia	0.96	5.50	–
2	54	pre	Endometrioid cystadenocarcinoma	Ia	0.64	0.96	–
3	46	pre	Borderline endometrioid cystadenocarcinoma	Ia	0.34	0.56	57
4	52	post	Serous cystadenocarcinoma	Ia	0.39	0.57	70
5	52	post	Serous cystadenocarcinoma	Ib	0.38	0.44	35
6	53	post	Endometrioid cystadenocarcinoma	Ic	0.58	0.80	26
7	30	pre	Borderline serous cystadenocarcinoma	Ia	0.43	0.59	15
8	37	pre	Serous cystadenocarcinoma	Ic	0.33	0.49	40
9	38	pre	Serous cystadenocarcinoma	IIa	0.41	0.56	32

RI, Resistance index; PI, pulsatility index; PSV, peak systolic velocity.

the cyst wall. It is easy in this situation to obtain a flow velocity waveform from an adjacent pelvic vessel that will probably have a notch in it. The location within a cyst of the area of blood flow detected by colour Doppler has also been given significance. If signals are recorded from septae or solid papillary projections, the cyst is more likely to be malignant. This rather misses the point that any lesion with septae and/or papillary projections is more likely to be malignant, irrespective of the colour Doppler findings. The data of Granberg et al. [16] confirm this (Figs. 1, 2).

Transvaginal colour Doppler findings must be looked at in the context of the patients history, the clinical appearances and the B-mode ultrasound findings. To expect that these blood flow data alone can be used to classify an ovarian cystic lesion is premature at this time. In our view, colour Doppler ultrasonography can be a useful part of the clinical evaluation of a patient, but should not be looked at in isolation. The bottom line with this argument is simple. What would be your actions if you found a 4.5-cm cyst with an irregular wall and several solid papillary projections, but no blood flow seen with colour Doppler? Would you be happy to reassure the women that she has no possibility of having ovarian cancer? I hope the answer would be no. Colour Doppler gives interesting insights into tumour pathology and a part of the diagnostic picture. However, it is still not clear whether it

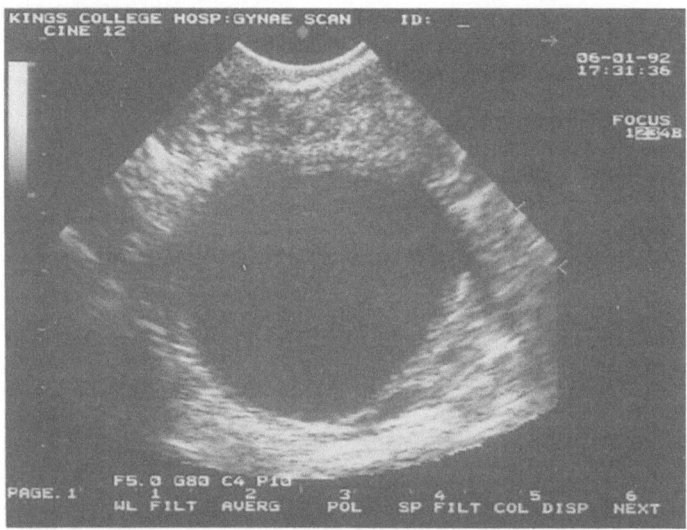

Fig. 1. A persistent simple unilocular cyst less than 5.0 cm in diameter. It is smooth walled, has hypoechogenic contents and has no papillary projections. Such a lesion is unlikely to be malignant

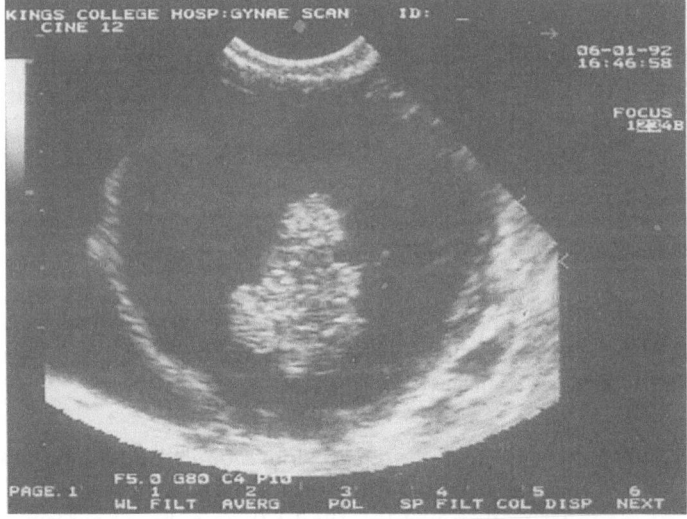

Fig. 2. A persistent unilocular cyst with an irregular papillary projection. This, coupled with the free fluid visible outside the ovary, indicates a high risk of malignancy

should be used in isolation to change the clinical management of patients. In view of this uncertainty, how can abnormal vascularity be defined according to colour and pulsed Doppler findings? Table 3 attempts to summarise our view of the situation.

Table 3. Indications of abnormal vascularity. *Note*: These indications can never be used in isolation. Other factors that Must be considered include menopausal status, ovarian cycle, pregnancy, drugs, history and finally the B-mode image

- From an area of morphological abnormality
- Persistent on repeat scan
- Characteristic flow velocity waveform
- Low impedance
- Relatively high velocity
- Take the "worst case" value, i.e. the point with the highest peak systolic velocity and lowest impedance
- Insufficient data to be categorical about cutoff values
- Qualitatively abnormal (i.e. the vessel pattern)

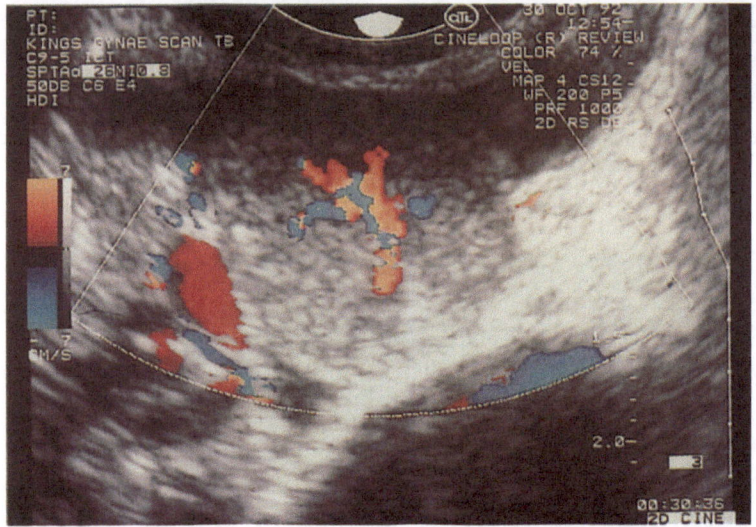

Fig. 3. A solid area of a stage II serous cystadenocarcinoma. A colour Doppler gate has been placed over the lesion and the pulsed repetition frequency (PRF) adjusted to detect low-velocity blood flow. A disordered branching pattern of blood vessels can be clearly seen. Such a vascular pattern seems more often associated with frequency malignancy

It is important to emphasise the need to use colour Doppler in a disciplined fashion, and its use within the strictly defined protocol of an ovarian cancer screening programme has been described [5]. Whilst there is broad agreement that low impedance is characteristic of carcinoma, the role of velocity measurements is less certain. This is important, as highly sensitive equipment will obtain low-impedance waveforms from almost any ovary (Bourne and Bauer 1995, unpublished data). These will invariably have a very low peak systolic velocity of less than 5 cm/s. It has certainly been our experience that cancers have been associated with higher peak systolic velocities (>10 cm/s) and tend to have a characteristic "whooshing" sound when listened to using pulsed

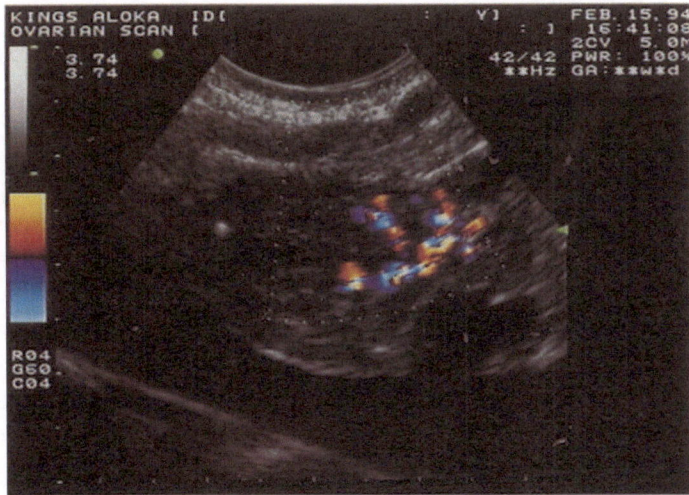

Fig. 4. Branching vessels within one section of an ovary containing a stage I serous cystadenocarcinoma. The cystic part of the lesion is not visible in this view because of the scanning plane adopted

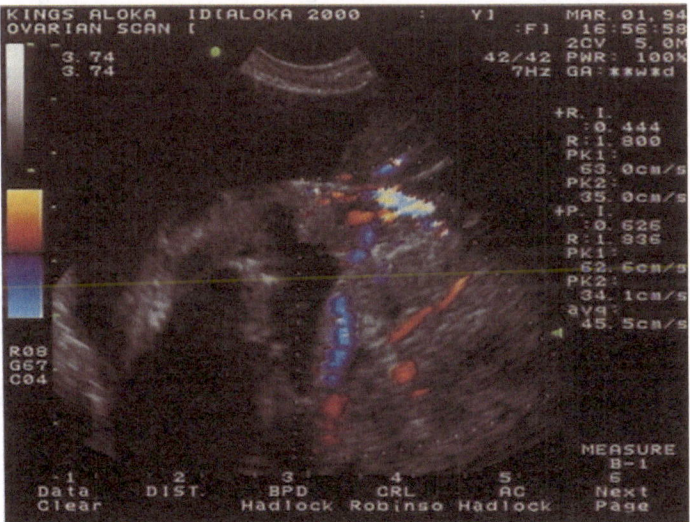

Fig. 5. Abundant florid vascularity within a solid portion of a stage III serous cystadeno-carcinoma

Doppler. Given the heterogeneous nature of ovarian malignancies, it seems sensible to record the "worst case" value for these indices of flow. In this way, sampling errors can be kept to a minimum. The qualitative appearance of the area of colour should also be assessed. Figures 3–5 demonstrate this feature.

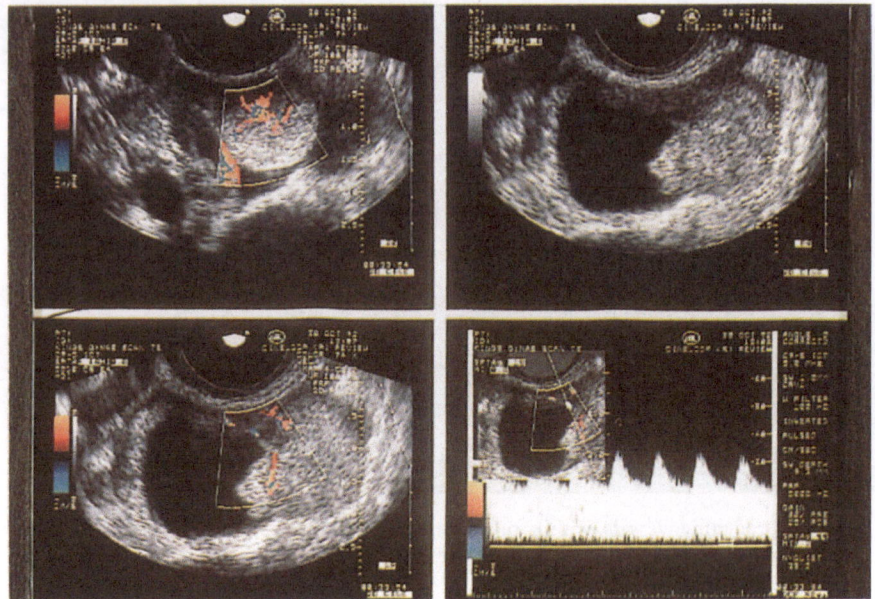

Fig. 6. A stage II serous cystadenocarcinoma (also see Fig. 3). All the criteria for malignancy are illustrated. The ovary is enlarged and contains an irregular cyst with solid papillary projections. There is florid vascularity with irregular branching vessels, and pulsed Doppler reveals low-impedance, relatively high velocity blood flow through the lesion. Although colour Doppler has added to the diagnostic picture, B-mode imaging alone would have led to the same management decisions being made with this patient had colour Doppler not been available

Branching areas of colour can be seen over the surface of these solid areas of tumour: a stage II (Fig. 3), stage I (Fig. 4) and stage III cystadenocarcinoma (Fig. 5). These lesions should be contrasted with Figs. 3 and 5 in the chapter on "Ovulation and the Periovulatory Follicle" by Bourne et al. In both cases the vascularity has a more ordered distribution. The vessels of the follicle are distributed evenly around the wall, whilst a ring of colour is formed around the solid corpus luteum.

Figure 6 shows a lesion that exemplifies the characteristics listed above for a malignant tumour. B-mode imaging reveals an enlarged ovary with abnormal morphology that persisted on repeat scan 6 weeks later. There is florid vascularisation visible using colour flow, and the vessels seen are branching and disordered (see Fig. 3). A pulsed Doppler range gate has been placed over the area of colour to reveal low-impedance, relatively high velocity blood flow through the ovary. It is important to note that the lesion had similar features at both the initial and repeat ultrasound scans. Histological examination of the lesion showed a stage II serous cystadenocarcinoma. The patient was asymptomatic and had a strong family history of both ovarian and breast cancer. She was 32 years old at the time of her diagnosis.

Finally, care must be taken not to extrapolate data from the examination of late-stage cancers to all ovarian cysts. There have been very few early stage cancers reported in the literature on which to base an opinion, although the majority of those described appear to demonstrate low-impedance blood flow [2, 22]. Conversely, with late stage disease, ischaemic changes within these tumours may also lead to an absence of obvious neovascularisation. Once again, clinicians must be aware of these potential limitations and never ignore either the B-mode image of a lesion or the overall clinical situation of the individual patient.

Ovarian Cancer Screening

Background

Ovarian cancer remains the most common cause of death from gynaecological malignancy. About 22 000 women in the United States develop the disease each year. In the early stages of the disease, there are few characteristic symptoms or signs, and as a result the majority of women with this disease present at stage III or IV, when palliation is often the only management strategy. The overall 5-year survival rate of less than 35% [25] is a reflection of the limited impact that new approaches to treatment have had on mortality from this disease. Conversely, the 5-year survival rate for women with stage I ovarian cancer may be over 90% [32]. In view of the depressing results relating to the treatment of late-stage disease, attempts are being made to develop effective screening procedures for early cancers in asymptomatic women. Once a test with suitable sensitivity and specificity for early-stage disease has been identified, a randomised trial will then need to be carried out to determine whether earlier diagnosis and treatment will improve the prognosis for substantially more women. The problems associated with ovarian cancer screening have been reviewed [4, 13].

The use of ultrasound to screen for ovarian cancer was first proposed by Campbell et al. in 1982 [9]. Subsequently, transabdominal ultrasound was used to screen over 5000 women for the presence of ovarian cancer in a large prospective trial [10]. This study suggests that whilst conventional transabdominal ultrasonography is a sensitive technique for the detection of small cystic lesions suggestive of cancer, it is difficult to discriminate between malignant and benign cystic lesions on the basis of transabdominal B-mode imaging alone. There are now reports on the use of higher resolution transvaginal ultrasound to screen for ovarian cancer both in normal [31] and high-risk populations [3]. The consensus view is that transvaginal ultrasonography is a sensitive first-stage screening test that will detect nearly all cystic ovarian lesions suggestive of carcinoma. What is needed is a second-stage test that will discriminate between benign and malignant cysts. Colour Doppler may have a role as a second-stage test, being used after an ovarian morphological abnormality has first been detected using B-mode imaging. In this context, the use of transvaginal colour Doppler has been used successfully to reduce the false-positive rate of ovarian cancer screening research programmes.

Table 4. The performance of different second stage tests in an ovarian cancer screening programme

	No second stage test	Unilocular or complex	Morphology score (MS)	Low PI (≤1.0)	Low PI or MS ≥ 5
DRate	100%	100%	83%	80%	100%
FPs	55 [13]	33 [nd]	6 [1]	13 [0]	15 [1]
Odds	1:9	1:6	1:1	1:3	2:5

DRate, detection rate; FPs, number of false positive test results; Odds, odds ratio of finding cancer at surgery; nd, No data available. Figures in brackets indicate postmenopausal women. Data derived from [6].

Screening Studies

Of particular interest are the data generated from the King's College Hospital familial ovarian cancer screening programme [6, 8]. A total of 1601 asymptomatic women with a family history of ovarian cancer were recruited to this study. Of these, 959 were pre-menopausal and so formed a particularly difficult group to examine; 157 women had a family pedigree consistent with site-specific ovarian cancer syndrome, and 288 with multiple site cancer syndrome (Lynch type II). The protocol and definition of a positive result have been described [3, 5]. A total of 61 women (3.8%) had a positive screen result (a persistent ovarian mass), six of whom had primary ovarian cancer detected at surgery (five stage Ia and one stage III). Second-stage tests were then used to try to discriminate between benign and malignant lesions. The use of a high morphological score or low-impedance blood flow increased the odds of finding cancer at surgery from 1:9 to about 2:5 (1:1 in the highest risk groups). It is worth studying these data in greater detail.

If all lesions in the study other than simple unilocular cysts had been removed, the number of false-positive test results would have been reduced by 40% from 55 to 33. The odds of finding cancer at surgery amongst women with a positive screen result would have been 1:6. If we had used a weighted morphology score (≥5), the false-positive rate would have been reduced by 89% from 55 to six. However, one cancer would have been missed. There would have been just one false-positive test result amongst the 469 postmenopausal women in the study, and the odds of finding an ovarian cancer at surgery would have been 1:1. Colour Doppler would have to perform very well to compare favourably to these figures. If the second-stage test had been based on finding a lesion with a PI of less than 1.0, the false-positive rate would have fallen 76% from 55 to 13. Twelve out of 13 of the false-positive test results would have occurred in women less than 53 years old. If we combine the two tests and say that any ovarian lesion with a morphology score of 5 or more or a PI of 1.0 or less must be treated as malignant, all the cancers would be detected, the number of false-positive test results would have been 15 and the odds of finding a cancer at surgery reduced to 2:5.

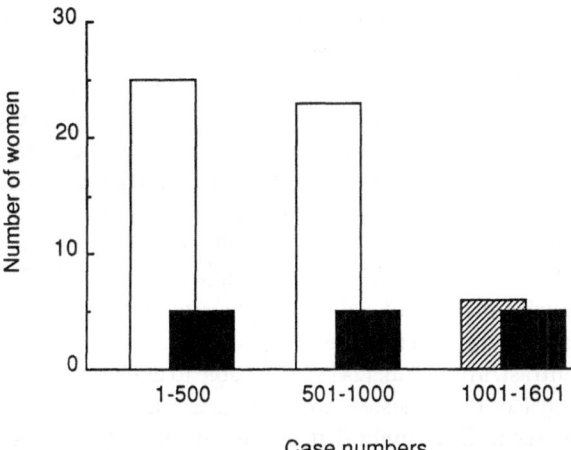

Fig. 7. The number of false-positive test results by screening number (from [6]). The use of combined second-stage tests prospectively performs as well as if they had been applied retrospectively. *White bars*, at first stage; *shaded bar*, after use of a high morphological score (MS; ≥5) or a low pulsatility index (PI) prospectively; *black bars*, after use of a high MS or a low PI retrospectively

The data showing the application of different second-stage tests in this ovarian cancer screening programme is summarised in Table 4. It is important to note that, because the study group is at increased risk of the disease, there is a prevalence effect. Hence the odds ratio is 1:9, even without a second-stage test. It is therefore arguable whether any other tests are necessary to reduce the false-positive rate when the risk of cancer is so high. If it is felt one is needed, a simple description of the cyst as being unilocular or complex will maintain 100% sensitivity, whilst reducing the number of false-positive test results by 33%; the odds ratio becomes 1:6. The use of a complicated morphology score significantly reduced the false-positive rate but at the expense of sensitivity (reduced to 83%), leaving an odds ratio of 1:1. As can be seen, using Doppler as a second-stage test results in a loss of sensitivity (80%); the number of false positive test results are reduced to 13 and the odds become 1:3. In this study, if these two assessments are combined such that either low-impedance flow or a high morphology score defined a positive result, a better test performance is obtained. As stated above, the detection rate is 100%, the number of false-positive test results 15 and the odds 2:5. The application of such a protocol either retrospectively or prospectively is shown in Fig. 7.

These data demonstrate that women with a strong family history of ovarian cancer are at increased risk of the disease and that transvaginal ultrasonography constitutes a sensitive first-stage test for its early detection. Given the prevalence effect, the use of any second stage tests in this group of women is debatable. Certainly in this study, colour Doppler performed less well than either a simple or complex evaluation of morphology. Only in combination with morphological information did it contribute significantly to overall test performance. Given that any screening test should be simple and reproducible, these data throw considerable doubt on the use of colour Doppler in this context. Doppler must perform at least as well or better than simpler, cheaper techniques if it is to find a clinical role in screening. It is interesting that the only other recent well-conducted studies reporting the results of a screening programme for familial ovarian cancer have also found that colour Doppler may have a limited role to play. Karlan et al. [18] studied 597 asymptomatic women with a family history of ovarian cancer. Low-impedance blood flow was observed within the ovaries of 80% of pre-menopausal women (n = 359) and 24% of women after the menopause (n = 36). This emphasises the need to restrict the use of colour Doppler within a screening algorithm to the role of a second-stage test; otherwise there may be a very high false-positive test rate. In contrast, Muto et al. [24] were unable to elicit satisfactory flow velocity waveforms in 40% of the persistent ovarian masses detected in their screening programme. There seems little doubt that, at the time of this writing, the currently available data do not justify the unguarded enthusiasm for the use of colour Doppler shown by some authors. The situation is not helped by the fact that few clinicians seem to understand the aims of screening or to be able to carry out their examinations within the confines of a strict protocol. There are no data relating to the use of transvaginal colour Doppler as a first-stage screening test for ovarian cancer, although it might be anticipated that the false-positive rate of such an approach would be unacceptable. Our current knowledge suggests that it can be used to add to the diagnostic information available about a persistent mass, its use confined to the role of a second-stage test. The real issue for the proponents of ovarian cancer screening is whether early detection actually alters the natural history of the disease and results in reduced mortality [7].

Further Potential Limitations and Prospects

Whilst it is not unreasonable to be optimistic, we must remember the potential limitations of colour Doppler. In post-menopausal women, there are no physiological events occurring within the ovary that may lead to altered vascularity. In our ovarian cancer screening programme, there have been very few false-positive results from post-menopausal women [6]. In pre-menopausal women, this is not the case. Similar processes of angiogenesis, and thus very similar indices of impedance to blood flow, are seen from within the developing corpus luteum and the pre-ovulatory follicle as are seen in early cancer (see previous chapters). Great care must therefore be taken to exclude vascular changes that are secondary to normal physiological events. Vascular information derived from the ovary must be viewed critically and related to the patient's ovarian cycle, and any abnormal findings subjected to a repeat scan. There is probably quite a narrow window within any ovarian cycle during which there will be a complete absence of angiogenic activity. Accordingly, for the purposes of ovarian cancer screening we currently examine pre-menopausal patients between days 3 and 11 of their cycle. If such a policy is adhered to, the majority of physiological lesions will be identified and false-positive test results avoided. However, it seems likely that low-impedance blood flow will be obtained from the majority of pre-menopausal ovaries. The dynamic nature of the ovaries in terms of both their vasculature and morphology must be appreciated. The uncritical enthusiasm of some authors for transvaginal colour Doppler is to be deprecated and is unhelpful to those of us who believe that this technique will improve our ability to diagnose early ovarian carcinoma. An unsigned editorial states that transvaginal colour Doppler can be used to detect ovarian cancer before it is otherwise discernible and that is should be utilised to characterise the nature of cystic ovarian lesions in pregnancy [23]. There are little data to support the former statement and none to support the latter. These problems have been discussed [11].

Despite these possible pitfalls transvaginal colour Doppler has already been shown to reduce the false-positive rate of an ultrasound-based screening programme [6]. Knowledge of the lesions likely to cause false-positive results with colour Doppler suggests that similar figures will be obtained when screening the general population. It has often been said that for a screening test for ovarian cancer to be credible, it would have to achieve a positive predictive value of better than 10% (an odds ratio of about 1:10); a combination of transvaginal ultrasonography and colour flow imaging satisfies this criteria. Any worries about colour Doppler findings in physiological lesions must be seen in the context of the technique being used as a second-stage test, its use being limited to persistent ovarian masses. Hence any mass found at screening would be subjected to a repeat scan at an interval, at which time colour Doppler would be performed. In this way most physiological lesions will have regressed. The fact that most cases of invasive stage I ovarian cancer examined using transvaginal colour Doppler have shown evidence of neovascularisation gives cause for optimism about the sensitivity of the test for early-stage disease. The sensitive way that colour Doppler detects vascular changes in the ovary around the time of ovulation suggests that if the development of new vessels is an obligate event in the earliest stages of ovarian cancer, colour Doppler will be able to demonstrate them. However, even in a high-risk population the prevalence of the disease means that about 300 women need to be screened in order to detect one case of early ovarian cancer. To examine the sensitivity and specificity of colour Doppler as a second-stage test in an ovarian cancer screening programme will require large-scale screening trials in order to have enough clinical material to work with. A prospective randomised trial is now required to satisfy this requirement as well as to answer the larger question of whether screening and hence early treatment will reduce the currently high mortality rate from this disease.

Outside screening, the reliable classification of persistent ovarian masses remains a challenge. The wide variability in results encountered by many users of colour Doppler has led to confusion. In fact colour Doppler is neither as good as some workers proclaim nor as bad as others would have us believe. The truth lies somewhere in the middle. Used uncritically, in isolation and in inexperienced hands, transvaginal colour Doppler will be at best useless and at worst dangerous. The number of doctors who wish to learn colour Doppler having had little or no experience of B-mode ultrasonography illustrate the problem. However, notwith-standing the limitations discussed in this chapter, when applied by expert opera-tors and in a disciplined fashion, it will add significantly to the diagnostic information available about both asymptomatic and symptomatic ovarian masses.

Acknowledgements. We are grateful to Keymed Ltd. (Southend, UK) and to the Aloka Co. Ltd. (Tokyo, Japan) for the use of their ultrasound equipment, and to Schering Health Care for their support of the gynaecological ultrasound clinic.

References

1. Bourne TH, Campbell S, Steer CV, Whitehead MI, Collins WP (1989) Transvaginal colour flow imaging: a possible new screening technique for ovarian cancer. Br Med J 299: 1367–1370
2. Bourne TH (1991) Transvaginal color Doppler in gynecology. Ultrasound Obstet Gynecol 1: 359–373
3. Bourne TH, Whitehead MI, Campbell S, Royston P, Bhan V, Collins WP (1991) Ultra-sound Screening for Familial Ovarian Cancer. Gynecol Oncol 43: 92–97
4. Bourne TH, Reynolds K, Campbell S (1991) Ovarian cancer screening. Eur J Cancer 27: 655–659
5. Bourne TH, Hampson J, Reynolds K, Collins WP, Campbell S (1992) Screening for early ovarian cancer. Br J Hosp Med 48: 454–459
6. Bourne TH, Campbell S, Reynolds KM, Whitehead MI, Hampson J, Royston P, Crayford TJB, Collins WP (1993) Screening for familial ovarian cancer with transvaginal ultrasonography and colour blood flow imaging. Br Med J 306: 1025–1029
7. Bourne TH (1993) Can ovarian masses be characterised using ultrasound? (Editorial.) Gynecol Oncol 51: 4–6
8. Bourne TH, Campbell S, Reynolds K, Hampson J, Bhatt L, Crayford TJB, Whitehead MI, Collins WP (1994) The potential role of serum CA 125 in an ultrasound-based screening program for familial ovarian cancer. Gynecol Oncol 52: 379–385
9. Campbell S, Goessens L, Goswamy R, Whitehead MI (1982) Real-time ultrasonography for determination of ovarian morphology and volume – a possible new screening test for early ovarian cancer? Lancet i: 425–426
10. Campbell S, Bhan V, Royston P, Whitehead MI, Collins WP (1989) Transabdominal ultrasound screening for early ovarian cancer. Br Med J 299: 1363–1367
11. Campbell S, Bourne TH, Collins WP (1990) Screening for ovarian cancer. Lancet 336: 436
12. Campbell S, Bourne TH, Reynolds K, Hampson J, Royston P, Whitehead MI, Collins WP (1991) Role of colour Doppler in an ultrasound based screening programme. In: Sharp F, Mason WP, Leake RE (eds) Ovarian cancer biological and therapeutic challenges II. Chapman and Hall Medical, Cambridge
13. Cuckle HS, Wald NJ (1990) The evaluation of screening tests for ovarian cancer. In: Sharp F, Mason WP, Leake RE (eds) Ovarian cancer: biological and therapeutic chal-lenges. Chapman and Hall Medical, Cambridge, pp 229–239
14. Fleischer AC, Williams LC, Jones HW III (1993) Transabdominal or transvaginal color Doppler sonography of ovarian massess. In: Fleischer AC, Jones HW III (eds) Early detection of ovarian cancer with transvaginal sonography: potentials and limitations. Raven, New York
15. Folkman J, Watson J, Ingber D, Hanahan D (1989) Induction of angiogenesis during the transition from hyperplasia to neoplasia. Nature 339: 58–61

16. Granberg S, Wikland M, Jansson I (1989) Macroscopic characterisation of ovarian tumors and the relation to the histological diagnosis: criteria to be used for ultrasound evaluation. Gynecol Oncol 35: 139–144
17. Hata K, Makihara K, Hata T, Takahashi K, Kitao M (1991) Transvaginal color Doppler imaging for haemodynamic assessment of tumors in the reproductive tract. Int J Gynecol Obstet 36: 301–308
18. Karlan BY, Raffel LJ, Crvenkovic G, Smrt C, Chen D, Lopez E, Walla CA, Garber C, Cane P, Sart DA, Rotter JI, Platt LD (1993) A multidisciplinary approach to the early detection of ovarian carcinoma: rationale, protocol design, and early results. Am J Obstet Gynecol 169: 494–501
19. Kurjak A, Zalud I, Jurkovic D, Alfirovic Z, Miljan M (1989) Transvaginal color flow Doppler for the assessment of pelvic circulation. Acta Obstet Gynecol Scand 68: 131–135
20. Kurjak A, Zalud I (1991) Early detection of ovarian cancer by transvaginal color Doppler. J Ultrasound Med 10: S57
21. Kurjak A, Zalud I, Alfirevic Z (1991) Evaluation of adnexal masses with transvaginal color ultrasound. J Ultrasound Med 10: 295–297
22. Kurjak A, Shalan R, Matijevic R, Predanic M, Kupesic-Urek S (1993) Stage I ovarian cancer by transvaginal color Doppler sonography: a report of 18 cases. Ultrasound Obstets Gynecol 3: 195–198
23. Lancet editorial (1990) First catch your deer. Lancet 336: 436
24. Muto MG, Cramer DW, Brown DL, Welsch WR, Harlow BL, Xu H, Brucks JP, Tsao S, Berkowitz RS (1993) Screening for ovarian cancer: the preliminary experience of a familial ovarian cancer center. Gynecol Oncol 51: 12–20
25. Petterson F (ed) (1991) Annual report on the results of treatment in gynecological cancer. Int J Gynecol Obstet 36 [Suppl]: 238–277
26. Ramos I, Fernanandez LA, Morse SS, Fortune KL, Taylor KJW (1988) Detection of neovascular signals in a 3 day walker rat carcinoma by CW Doppler ultrasound. Ultrasound Med Biol 14: 123–126
27. Rastinejad F, Polverini PJ, Bouck NP (1985) Regulation of the activity of a new inhibitor of angiogenesis by a cancer suppressor gene. Cell 56: 345–355
28. Reynolds K, Campbell S, Maghaddam A, Lawton F, Bourne TH, Farzaneh F, Collins W, Harris AL, Bicknell R (1994) Correlation of ovarian malignancy with expression of platelet-derived endothelial growth factor. J Natl Cancer Inst 86: 1234–1238
29. Shimamoto K, Sakuma S, Ishigaki T, Makino N (1987) Intratumoral blood flow; evaluation with colour Doppler echography. Radiology 165: 683–685
30. Tekay A, Jouppila A (1992) Validity of pulsatility and resistance indices in classification of adnexal tumors with transvaginal color Doppler ultrasound. Ultrasound Obstet Gynecol 2: 338–344
31. Van Nagell JR, De Priest PD, Puls LE, Donaldson ES, Gallion HH, Paulik EJ, Powell DE, Kryscio PJ (1991) Ovarian cancer screening in asymptomatic women by transvaginal sonography. Cancer 68: 458–462
32. Young RC, Walton LA, Ellenberg SS, Homesley HD, Wilbanks GD, Decker DG, Miller A, Park R, Major F Jr (1990) Adjuvant therapy in stage I and stage II epithelial ovarian cancer – results of two prospective randomised trials. N Engl J Med 322: 1021–1027

Transvaginal Color Doppler Ultrasound in Pelvic Inflammatory Disease

M. Toth and F.A. Chervenak

Pelvic inflammatory disease (PID) is infection of the female upper genital tract. It is the most serious complication of sexually transmitted bacterial diseases. Because of the wide variety of adverse effects on reproductive performance, PID will have a negative physical and emotional impact on the woman's life.

The major sequelæ of PID are infertility, ectopic pregnancy, and chronic pelvic pain [1]. It is estimated that, in the United States, 10%–15% of women of reproductive age have had at least one episode of PID, and each year close to 1 000 000 new cases develop. About 30% of infertility and 50% of ectopic pregnancies are caused by PID. Every year about 50 000 operations are performed for which PID is the primary indication. Nearly 40 000 ectopic pregnancies each year are attributed to PID. Only about one half of women who have had even one instance of PID can subsequently become pregnant after these ectopic pregnancies [2, 3]. In addition, there is new evidence to suggest that subsequent pregnancies following PID have an increased incidence of adverse outcome [4].

Sexually active adolescents are at the greatest risk for PID. Other risk factors include multiple sex partners, a high number of sex partners throughout life, use of an intrauterine device (IUD), untreated infected male sex partner(s), a history of previous PID, presence of *Neisseria gonorrhoeae* or chlamydia in the reproductive tract, and frequent vaginal douching [1].

PID results in more morbidity than necessary for three major reasons: (1) women are not hospitalized when they should be, (2) many women receive inadequate or inappropriate antibiotic therapy, and (3) the male sex partner is not treated or is treated inadequately. PID is thought of as by many specialists as "the most neglected disease in the United States today."

Pathogenesis

In most cases of PID the infection is ascending and polymicrobial. Other less common routes of infection are hematogenous (mycoplasmas, mycobacteria) or by direct extension from an other abdominal organ (diverticulitis, appendicitis). The most commonly isolated anaerobic bacteria in PID are *Bacteroides* species and *Peptostreptococci*. Several different aerobic and anaerobic bacteria are present in the cervix, uterus, or the tubes. Among the sexually transmitted pathogens, *Neisseria gonorrhoeae* and *Chlamydia trachomatis* are most commonly identified.

The mechanism leading to tubal damage seems to be different in gonococcal and chlamydial salpingitis. In vitro experiments have shown that *Neisseria gonorrhoeae* elicited more serious damage to tubal tissue than did *Chlamydia trachomatis*. This was due to the direct effect of the bacterium on the ciliated epithelial cells. The reverse is true in vivo [5].

A complicated immunological process is thought to be responsible for most of the scar tissue formation in women infected with chlamydia. Present in 60%–70% of cases, this bacterium has evolved as the most important and most common pathogen of PID. Its 57-kDa membrane protein is a member of the 60-kDa family of heat shock proteins. These highly antigenic proteins are present in many bacteria and also in several eukaryotic organisms, including man. Chlamydial heat shock proteins are capable of sensitizing human T lymphocytes [6]. Because the human and chlamydial heat shock proteins are about 50% homologous, lymphocytes that were sensitized by chlamydia can also respond to human heat shock protein, which is released by the host cells under environmental stress. The end result is a delayed autoimmune hypersensitivity reaction, which continues to cause progressive damage even after the elimination of chlamydia. This phenomenon will also increase the severity of tissue damage after repeated exposure to the organism [7]. In our experience, 50% of women who developed lymphocyte sensitization to chlamydia heat shock protein had had at least two episodes of PID. Only early recognition and aggressive treatment will prevent the immune system from becoming activated.

Prevention

Once PID develops, it has an unpredictable effect on the reproductive performance of the woman. Therefore, the best way to deal with PID at present is to prevent it. This can be accomplished by educating the population at risk in sexual practices and identifying and treating the asymptomatic infectious male population, which is most often responsible for the spread of this disease.

Symptoms and Diagnosis

More than half of women with PID will develop tubal damage without any symptoms of the disease. These cases are most commonly associated with chlamydia infection. Because of this new observation, the Centers for Disease Control recently suggested the following new classifications for this disease:

1. *Silent (asymptomatic) PID.* Tubal scarring occurs without the patient's knowledge. The first contact with these women is as the time of their work-up for tubal factor infertility.
2. *Atypical PID.* Patients have minimal symptoms only, consisting of midcycle bleeding, spotting, irregular periods, and mild low abdominal discomfort.

3. *Acute PID.* This form is most commonly seen in patients presenting to emergency rooms throughout the country. These women are acutely ill, have moderate to severe low abdominal pain, cervical motion tenderness, adnexal swelling, and tenderness and usually heavy vaginal and urethral discharge.
4. *PID residual syndrome.* This group of patients have the end result of the disease with chronic pelvic pain and scar tissue formation.

Laparoscopy is the diagnostic procedure of choice for establishing or excluding a diagnosis based on visual evidence of pelvic inflammation. About 20% of women with laparoscopically proven salpingitis will have classic symptoms of PID [8].

It is estimated that about two thirds of women with PID can be identified based on clinical symptoms only. Bacterial identification was greatly aided by the invention of polymerase chain reaction (PCR) technology, which is capable of amplifying bacterial DNA [9]. In a small study of women with high-risk sexual behavior, we found PCR ten times more sensitive than regular chlamydia culture. The more recently introduced ligand chain reaction test (LCR) offers so far the best results in chlamydia detection. Its accuracy on cervical specimens is somewhat better than that of the PCR method and it can also be used on semen and urine.

LCR will be the choice of large screening studies in the future. Tumor necrosis factor (TNF)-α_a cytokine produced by macrophages is usually elevated in the infected tubal tissue of women with PID [10]. Its measurement may help to confirm or to rule out upper genital tract infection. Recently we succeeded in developing a lymphocyte proliferation assay to chlamydia heat shock protein. It also correlated well with upper genital tract infection [11]. Other, less specific, blood tests include estimated sedimentation rate and C-reactive protein measurements. Both have very low predictive values.

Ultrasound has been gaining acceptance in the diagnosis of PID. With a transvaginal method utilizing gray scale imaging, Patten successfully diagnosed inflammation in 25 of 27 cases [12]. From our experience, adding color to the ultrasound image improves visualization of both the normal and the abnormal structures. In addition, because the inflammatory process involves both structural and vascular changes, we have introduced color Doppler ultrasound as an adjunct to imaging.

Ovarian Blood Flow in Women with Pelvic Inflammatory Disease

Many studies have been undertaken to assess blood flow-related functional changes in the ovaries. For example, color Doppler was used to study follicular morphology and flow patterns in the periovulatory period. Significant changes in resistance to flow have been described in the active ovary. Most of these changes were attributed to angiogenesis in the corpus luteum [13, 14]. Moreover, ovarian blood flow was studied longitudinally during the entire menstrual cycle of infertile patients and normal controls by Kurjak et al. [15]. Infertile patients were found to have increased resistance to flow in the active ovary when compared to controls. Kurjak et al. [16] and Bourne et al. [17] have pioneered the use of transvaginal color Doppler to assess pelvic blood flow in different pathologies, including ovarian malignancy. Bourne et al. [17] and Kurjak et al. [18] used this method to measure blood flow impedance in ovarian tumors to screen for malignancy. Examining a large number of two different sets of women, both groups of investigators were successful in identifying cases of ovarian cancer at an early stage.

We believed that ovarian blood flow may be affected by an inflammatory process in the pelvis. This hypothesis was based on two premises: (1) that the ovary is in close proximity to the tube which is the primary focus of infection in PID and (2) because of its anatomic location, the ovary shares a significant part of its blood supply with the ipsilateral tube. It is relatively easy to identify the ovaries, especially in young women.

The normal ovarian volume is, in women of reproductive age, in the range of 4–6 cm^3. Tubal visualization, however, requires an experienced sonologist. Unless there is fluid collection in the lumen or in the peritoneal cavity, it will be difficult to visualize even parts of the fallopian tubes [19]. The ovary receives its blood supply from the ovarian and the uterine arteries. These vessels reach the ovary through the infundibulopelvic and ovarian ligaments. They anastomose alongside the ovary and give off numerous small branches into the mesosalpinx to supply the tube. These arteries can readily be identified by color Doppler ultrasound [12]. Ovarian parenchymal blood flow can be obtained easily both from the active and the inactive ovary late in the follicular phase. In our experience, the resistance in the parenchymal blood vessels varies in the acute phase of PID, but it is almost invariably increased in the more advanced stage, when some degree of tissue damage has already developed.

In a study of 42 women with suspected PID, we performed color Doppler ultrasound prior to the diagnostic laparoscopy. Fourteen patients had normal pelvic findings or other pathology. The remaining 28 women had PID with some degree of permanent tissue damage in all cases (PID residual syndrome). The intraovarian resistance was found to be increased in all but two patients, as indicated by a higher pulsatility index (PI) with a range of 0.9–2.8. The PI in the controls ranged between 0.4 and 1.1. The difference was statistically significant. No acute PID cases were included in this group [19].

In another observation of six women with primary infertility, four had laparoscopically proven permanent tubal damage caused by infection (silent PID). They all had a PI of more than 1.5 [19]. The measurements were taken in the follicular phase between days 9–12 of the cycle because of the obvious effect of the corpus luteum on ovarian compliance. In cases of acute PID, we found that the ovarian resistance indices varied between nondetectable and high-resistance values. This phenomenon is probably attributable to the rapid pathological changes that occur within the infected organ. As infection develops, the increased blood flow and tissue swelling may result in a pressure increase in the encapsulated ovary. The less elastic capsule may resist parenchymal swelling, which results in increased intraparenchymal pressure and a greater resistance index. In the chronic cases, scar tissue formation is most likely responsible for the increased resistance. It was interesting to note that, in many cases, the flow indices returned to normal after treatment. Large prospective studies are needed to further assess the role of ovarian blood flow measurements in the diagnosis of different pelvic pathologies.

Acute Pelvic Inflammatory Disease

There is a characteristic way that the detectable signs appear on transvaginal sonogram during the course of PID. Early on, the sonographic findings may be entirely normal, except for fluid collection in the pelvis or in the uterine cavity. The latter may be the only sign of endometritis. As the infection progresses, an increased number of changes can occur in the pelvic organs with characteristic sonographic features [20]. Visualization of the fallopian tubes greatly improves the accuracy of the diagnosis. Because their echogenecity is the same as that of the surrounding organs, the normal tubes are hard to visualize by sonogram unless there is a significant fluid accumulation in the pelvis [21].

Hyperemia, swelling, tortuosity, and purulent exudate from the lumen and the serosal surfaces of the tubes are the main characteristics of acute PID. Of twelve women with laparoscopically proven acute salpingitis, by ultrasound we were able to identify fluid collection in the lumen of one or both tubes in ten cases within 72 h following onset of the symptoms.

The exudate is usually seen within the lumen of the ampullary portion of the tube. This is the area in which permanent tubal damage most commonly develops and in which ectopic pregnancies most commonly occur.

Using a novel approach in a prospective study of 26 women with acute PID, we successfully removed the tubal exudate with antibiotic lavage. A 2-mm ballooned catheter was inserted into the uterine cavity, the balloon was inflated, and a mixture of vibromycin and cefoxitin solution was injected into the uterus. Transvaginal color Doppler ultrasound was used to monitor the flow through the tubes into the abdominal cavity. The more fluid accumulated in the pelvis, the easier tubal visualization became. There were no complications. However, most patients required some pain medication. The clinical symptoms of acute PID seemed to resolve much faster in patients who underwent this procedure.

At 6 months follow-up, all 26 patients had bilateral tubal patency proven by hysterosalpingography. Ten of the 26 women were sensitized to chlamydia heat shock protein, a condition which carries a very high risk for permanent tubal damage. Eleven women who were sensitized to heat shock protein, but did not have tubal lavage, were used as controls. At 6 months follow-up, seven control patients were found to have developed unilateral or bilateral tubal blockage. It seems from the study that tubal lavage shortens recovery and preserves tubal patency in patients with PID.

Tubal swelling was documented in all patients, as represented by an ampullary diameter of greater than 10 mm. Blood vessels in the tubal wall are easily identified by color Doppler in this early phase of the disease. The ovaries are enlarged, globular, and they may contain multiple cysts. The cysts are infected follicles. The margins may be indistinct due to the accompanying perioophoritis. We found no characteristic changes in resistance indices of the uterine and ovarian arteries of women with acute salpingitis. Intraovarian parenchymal blood flow indices, however, varied between low and slightly elevated values (PI, 0.4–1.5).

Tuboovarian Abscess

Tuboovarian abscess (TOA) is the most severe form of acute infection. The continuous spillage of purulent material from the tube reaches the ovarian surface and neighboring structures (bowel, omentum). The end result is a complex adnexal conglomerate with a hypoechoic, septate sonographic appearance. The initial impression is that of a solid mass, but the acoustic enhancement and the total absence of blood flow confirms the presence of complex fluid. The external margins are irregular and indistinct. Sometimes it is difficult to identify the ovary or tube within the mass. The tube may be dilated and partially filled with fluid, as shown by the fluid debris levels. Part of the mass may appear in the cul-de-sac, which contains echogenic pus as well.

The more advanced the disease, the more ill-defined the TOA becomes, with complete loss of anatomic landmarks. The full extent of the process at this point is best determined by transabdominal ultrasound [22]. The abscess cavities can be safely drained under sonographic guidance. This procedure usually enhances recovery. Periappendiceal and diverticular abscess, endometriomas, benign and malignant ovarian tumors, and ectopic pregnancy have to be considered in the differential diagnosis. Chronic pelvic inflammatory disease (PID residual syndrome) can develop as a consequence of an acute infection or even in patients without any clinical evidence of salpingitis. The obstruction of the fimbriated end results in fluid collection in the tube, thus producing hydrosalpinx. This is a tubular anechoic structure on sonogram. The absence of blood flow on color Doppler helps differentiate the hydrosalpinx from a large blood vessel. Thickened mucosal folds and nodular projections into the lumen are characteristic sonographic signs. The appearance of internal echoes in the distended lumen with absence of blood flow suggests pyosalpinx. The adjacent ovary may be recognized with its convex border slightly compressing the wall of the anechoic fluid-filled hydrosalpinx. Loss of mobility in the different pelvic organs can occur because of extensive adhesions. The ovarian parenchymal blood flow is almost invariably decreased, as indicated by elevated PI values. The ovarian volume is normal or increased.

References

1. Expert Committee on Pelvic Inflammatory Disease (1991) Research directions for the 1990s. Sex Trans Dis 18: 46–64
2. Gales W, Wasserheit JN (1991) Genital chlamydial infections: epidemiology and reproductive sequelae. Am J Obstet Gynecol 164: 1771–1781
3. Toth M, Chaundray A, Witkin SS. Pregnancy outcome following pelvic infection. Infec Dis Obstet Gynecol (in press)
4. Weström L (1980) Incidence, prevalence and trends of acute pelvic inflammatory disease and its consequences in industrialized countries. Am J Obstet Gynecol 138: 880–892
5. Battiger BE, Frair J, Newhall WV, Katz BP (1989) Association of recurrent chlamydial infection with gonorrhea. J Infec Dis 159: 661–669
6. Morrison RP, Manning DS, Caldwell MD (1992) Immunology of chlamydia trachomatis infection: immunoprotective and immunopathogenetic responses. Adv Host Defense Mech 8: 57–84
7. Morrison RP, Bellard RJ, Lyng K, Caldwell HD (1989) Chlamydia disease pathogenesis. The 57 KD chlamydial hypersensitivity antigen is a stress response protein. J Exp Med 170: 1271–1283
8. Sellors J, Mahony J, Goldsmith C, Rath D (1991) The accuracy of clinical findings and laparoscopy in pelvic inflammatory disease. Am J Obstet Gynecol 164: 113–120
9. Bobo L, Coutle F, Yollken RH, Quinn T, Viscichi RP (1990) Diagnosis of chlamydia trachomatis cervical infection by detection of amplified DNA with a unique immunoassay. J Clin Microbiol 28: 1968–1973
10. Toth M, Jeramias J, Ledger WJ, Witkin SS (1992) In vivo tumor necrosis factor production in women with salpingitis. Surg Gynecol Obstet 174: 359–362
11. Witkin SS, Toth M, Jeremias J, Ledger WJ (1991) Increased inducability of inflammatory mediators from peripheral blood neuronuclear cells of women with salpingitis. Am J Obstet Gynecol 165: 719–723
12. Schotter MEW, Wladimiroff J, van Rijen HJM, Hop WCJ (1989) Uterine and ovarian flow velocity waveforms in the normal menstrual cycle: transvaginal Doppler study. Fertil Steril 52: 981–985
13. Collins WP, Jurkovič D, Bourne TH, Kurjak A, Campbell S (1991) Ovarian morphology, endocrine function and intrafollicular blood flow during the peri-ovulatory period. Human Reprod 6: 319–329
14. Fleischer A, Mckee MS, Gordon AN, et al (1990) Transvaginal sonography of postmenopausal ovaries with pathologic correlation. J Ultrasound Med 9: 637
15. Kurjak A, Schulman H, et al (1991) Transvaginal color flow Doppler in the assessment of ovarian and uterine blood flow in infertile women. Fertil Steril 56: 870–873
16. Kurjak A, et al (1989) Transvaginal color ultrasound for the assessment of pelvic circulation. Acta Obstet Gynecol Scand 68: 131–135
17. Bourne TH, Campbell S, Steer CH, et al (1989) Transvaginal color flow imaging: a possible new screening technique for ovarian cancer. Br Med J 299: 1367–1370
18. Kurjak A, Zalud I, Alferevic Z (1991) Evaluation of adnexal masses with transvaginal color Doppler ultrasound. J Ultrasound Med 10: 295–297
19. Toth M, Chervenak FA, Witkin SS, Ledger WJ (1992) Color Doppler ultrasound in the diagnosis of pelvic inflammatory disease. Annual meeting of the Infectious Diseases Society for Obstetrics and Gynecology, San Diego (abstr 7)
20. Patten RM, Vincent LM, Wolner-Hanssen P, Thorpe E Jr (1990) Pelvic inflammatory disease: endovaginal sonography with laparoscopic correlation. J Ultrasound Med 9: 681–689
21. Timor-Tritsch IE, Rottem S (1987) Transvaginal ultrasonographic study of the Fallopian tube. Obstet Gynecol 70: 424–428
22. Spirtos NJ, Bernstein RL, Crawford WL, Fayle J (1982) Sonography in acute pelvic inflammatory disease. J Reprod Med 6: 312–319

Transvaginal Colour Doppler Studies of Ectopic Pregnancy

D. Jurkovic, E. Jauniaux, and S. Campbell

Introduction

The diagnosis of early pregnancy and its abnormalities has been much improved by the advent of transvaginal ultrasonography. This technique has proved to be particularly useful for the assessment of patients who may have an ectopic pregnancy [19, 21]. The use of transvaginal rather than transabdominal probes increases both the sensitivity and specificity of the procedure [24]. Furthermore, it is possible in most cases to make a positive diagnosis based on the direct observation of an ectopic sac or adnexal mass [4]. In addition, an intra-uterine pregnancy can be detected earlier than by abdominal scanning.

However, in patients with suspected ectopic pregnancies, non-diagnostic ultrasound findings are found in 9%–37% of cases [5, 8]. The proportion of inconclusive results is greatest in the group of patients with abnormal intra-uterine pregnancy, in which the diagnosis cannot be reached in 21% of patients. An abnormal adnexal mass can be seen in about 90% of patients with surgically proven ectopics [19], although some have recently reported detection rates as low as 47% [17]. The presence of the embryo or yolk-sac within the adnexal mass provides certain diagnosis of ectopic pregnancy in 60%–70% of cases. In the remaining patients, the appearance of ectopic pregnancies is non-specific and often difficult to distinguish from chronic tubal damage or corpus luteum cyst. This can also lead to false-positive diagnosis of ectopic pregnancy in patients with other pelvic pathology. False-positive diagnoses are made in 5% of patients, and in most cases unusual appearances of a corpus luteum cyst were the cause of diagnostic errors [24].

In this chapter we will describe transvaginal colour Doppler findings in patients with ectopic pregnancies. Information obtained by blood flow studies helps to overcome some of the problems described above and increases the diagnostic accuracy of ultrasound in both abnormal intrauterine and ectopic pregnancies.

Characteristics of Blood Flow in Ectopic Pregnancies

The recent introduction of transvaginal pulsed and colour Doppler has facilitated studies of blood flow in pelvic vessels. The major advantage of colour Doppler is that blood flow can be displayed simultaneously with the conventional B-mode image [13]. This facility enables an assessment to be made of blood flow character-istics in small vascular branches, which are more difficult to detect by the tradi-tional pulsed Doppler technique. The use of colour Doppler to determine blood flow characteristics in the developing corpus luteum and in the main uterine, radial and spiral arteries in normal intra-uterine pregnancies at 4–18 weeks gesta-tion has been described [2, 10] (see chapter by Jauniaux et al. on "Transvaginal Colour Doppler Investigation of the Utero-Placental Circulation").

The terminal part of the uterine arterial circulation, the spiral arteries, are visualized by colour Doppler as a neovascular area immediately below the pla-centa. Flow velocity waveforms can be obtained from the spiral arteries by pulsed Doppler and impedance to flow analyzed by using the pulsatility or resistance index. Blood flow in an ectopic pregnancy can be examined in a similar way [22]. Colour Doppler is used first to demonstrate the vascular supply to the ectopic pregnancy. Once an area of neovascularity at the periphery of the sac is identified, the examination is completed using pulsed Doppler (Fig. 1).

In normal pregnancies there is a progressive decrease in impedance to flow in the main uterine artery and spiral arteries with gestational age. A decrease in impedance is accompanied by increased blood flow velocity in the main uterine artery. These findings are indirect evidence of a major increase in blood supply to meet the demand of the developing conceptus [10]. Regulation of this process is not fully understood, but it seems that hormonally mediated vasodilatation [20] and progressive trophoblastic invasion play major roles [18].

The Corpus luteum can be localized in all patients during the first 9 weeks of pregnancy by using colour Doppler. Even in patients with solid corpora lutea which cannot be identified on B-mode scan, colour Doppler will demonstrate typical areas of high vascularity with low resistance to blood flow (Fig. 2). Imped-ance to flow in the corpus luteum does not change during the first trimester in spite of significant variations in its hormonal production. This finding is in agreement with the hypothesis of different mechanisms of blood flow regulation to the corpus luteum compared to the vasculature in other hormone-responsive tissues [25]. Vessels in the corpus luteum originate from a process of neo-angiogenesis that

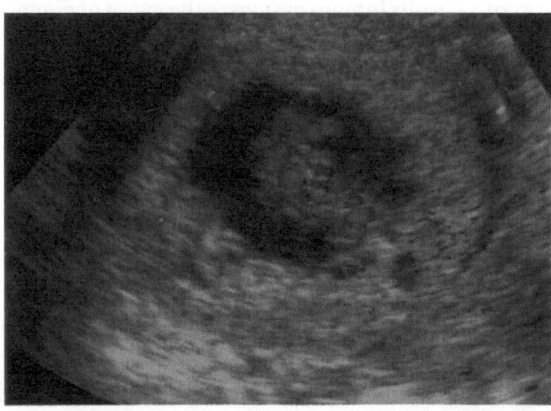

Fig. 1. Colour Doppler find-ings in a patient with a tubal ectopic sac and live embryo. Note the presence of blood flow at the periphery of the sac and within the placenta

starts around the time of the luteinizing hormone (LH) surge [6]. In some species there is a lack of muscular elements in the vessel walls and an absence of any autonomic innervation [3]. These immature vessels are probably incapable either of dilatation or constriction. Therefore, the type of circulation in the corpus luteum resembles to some extent the circulation in neoplastic tissues. These circulatory changes seem to be dissociated from the endocrine function of the corpus luteum.

Analysis of blood flow in patients with ectopic pregnancies and an obvious adnexal mass on transvaginal scan shows many similarities to those described in normal intra-uterine pregnancies. This similarity occurs in the presence of heterogeneity in the morphological findings, including cases of viable pregnancy and tubal abortion. In both main uterine arteries impedance to flow decreases and the calculated resistance index values are well within the reference ranges for normal intra-uterine pregnancy. However, uterine blood flow velocity is lower in the ectopic group, indicating an overall reduction in uterine blood supply [11]. This reduction may be the consequence of a reduced mass of viable trophoblast or perhaps a larger contribution from the ovarian arteries to the blood supply of tubal pregnancy. The lack of significant differences in blood flow parameters between the contralateral uterine arteries supports the hypothesis of a predominance of hormonal events in regulating blood flow in these vessels, as opposed to a local reduction in flow impedance caused by placentation.

Blood flow in the tubal branches of the uterine artery may be affected by the site of an ectopic sac. Kirchler et al. [12] have found significantly lower impedance to flow in the tubal arterial branch on the side of ectopic sac compared to the artery on the other side. However, in a few patients with a corpus luteum on the contralateral side to the ectopic, resistance to flow was lower on the side of the corpus luteum. Therefore, it remains unclear whether the increase in blood flow is caused primarily by the presence of active trophoblast or a corpus luteum.

An area of high vascularity at the periphery of the adnexal mass can be found in 94% ectopic pregnancies. The appearance and location of blood flow in relation

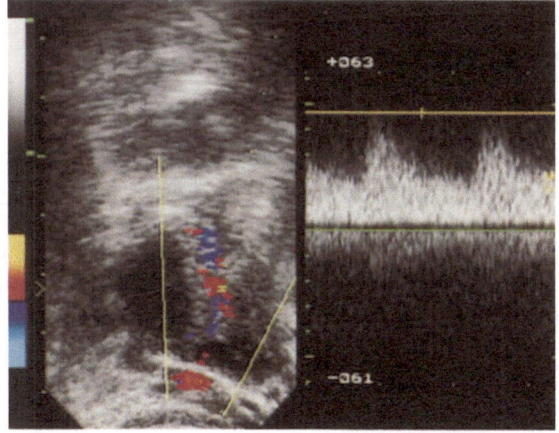

Fig. 2. Vascular supply to the corpus luteum. Typical low-impedance flow velocity waveforms are obtained by pulsed Doppler

to the gestational sac and the flow velocity waveform characteristics are similar to those obtained from the spiral arteries in normal intra-uterine pregnancies. However, the decrease in the impedance to flow with gestation observed in normal intra-uterine pregnancies does not occur in the ectopic group.

Histological studies have shown that in tubal gestations the development of the placenta replicates that seen in intra-uterine pregnancies [16]. Invasion of maternal blood vessels within the tube also occurs in the same way as in the uterus. Although the structure of vessels in the tubal wall differs markedly from that of the spiral arteries, the sequence of changes is similar. Therefore, it is not surprising that Doppler characteristics of the vascular supply to the gestational sac are almost identical in patients with intra-uterine or extra-uterine pregnancy. This finding applies to both the appearance and location of flow at the periphery of the sac and the flow velocity waveform characteristics. However, there is a subjective impression that the number of arterial branches supplying the sac was smaller in ectopic pregnancies compared to the number of the uterine spiral arteries, particularly in cases of tubal abortions.

Colour Doppler enables the detection of the corpus luteum in all women with an ectopic pregnancy [11]. In most cases it is located on the same side as the ectopic sac. Characteristics of blood flow as defined by colour and pulsed Doppler are identical in intra-uterine and ectopic pregnancy. Comparisons between ectopic and normal pregnancies paired for human chorionic gonadotrophin (hCG) concentration at 7–8 weeks gestation have shown lower levels of serum oestradiol and progesterone in ectopic pregnancies [9]. Although these findings suggest some degree of luteal insufficiency in ectopic pregnancy, recent data have shown that a luteo-placental shift in steroid synthesis occurs before 7 weeks gestation [7]. Therefore, it is more likely that decreased hormonal production reflects a reduction in the viability of the trophoblastic tissue. Lack of any differences in corpus luteum blood flow impedance between the two groups in our study supports this hypothesis. In view of apparent dissociation between endocrine function and blood supply to the corpus luteum, it is impossible to predict at this stage how useful blood flow studies may be for the assessment of its function in pregnancy.

Role of Colour Doppler in the Diagnosis and Management of Ectopic Pregnancy

The impact of colour Doppler on the diagnosis of ectopic pregnancy has been evaluated in a few recent reports. Pellerito et al. [15] have found that Doppler information greatly increases detection rate of the adnexal mass in patients with clinical suspicion of ectopic pregnancy. The sensitivity of 54% with B-mode imaging alone increased to 95% with the use of colour flow imaging. Similar results were reported by Emerson et al. [8], who found an increase in sensitivity from 71% to 87%. However, in both studies the detection rate of ectopic pregnancy by B-mode transvaginal scan were well below the expected standard rate of 80%–90%, which makes interpretation of their results difficult.

There are also differences in reported blood flow detection rates in patients with surgically confirmed ectopic pregnancies. We have found blood flow at the periphery of the ectopic trophoblast in 18 out of 19 (94%) cases [11]. Similar results were reported by Kurjak et al. [14], who detected blood flow in 88% of patients with ectopic pregnancies. However, Tekay and Jouppila [23] were able to obtain clear blood signals only in 50% of ectopic pregnancies. These differences can be partly explained by the large number of complex adnexal masses in the last study, which indicate tubal abortion and poor viability of trophoblast. Comparisons with hormone levels showed poor ectopic blood flow in patients with β-hCG levels below 100 mIU/ml (First International Reference Preparation). It has been suggested that the absence of blood flow can be used to select the patients who may benefit from conservative management. It is believed that the risk of tubal rupture should be lower with poor perfusion, but further studies are needed to confirm this.

Colour Doppler enables the diagnosis of ectopic pregnancy to be made in cases where appearances are non-specific. This is particularly useful in patients with an empty sac or solid ectopic. The demonstration of a characteristic blood flow distribution and signals enables definite diagnosis, something which is impossible to achieve by B-mode imaging alone (Fig. 3). However, corpus luteum blood flow has to be identified separately from ectopic flow in all cases to avoid false-positive diagnoses. If this cannot be achieved, it is more likely that an unusual-looking adnexal mass represents the corpus luteum rather than an ectopic pregnancy (Fig. 4).

Blood flow studies are particularly useful in patients with an abnormal intra-uterine pregnancy who are referred for an ultrasound scan to exclude ectopic pregnancy. As mentioned before, the number of inconclusive findings is greatest in this group. In up to 94% of patients who miscarry there is no visible intra-uterine sac, which adds to the uncertainty of the diagnosis. The demonstration of a typical trophoblastic blood supply increases the diagnostic sensitivity from 24% to 59% [8] (Fig. 5). Bearing in mind that the majority of patients with suspected ectopic

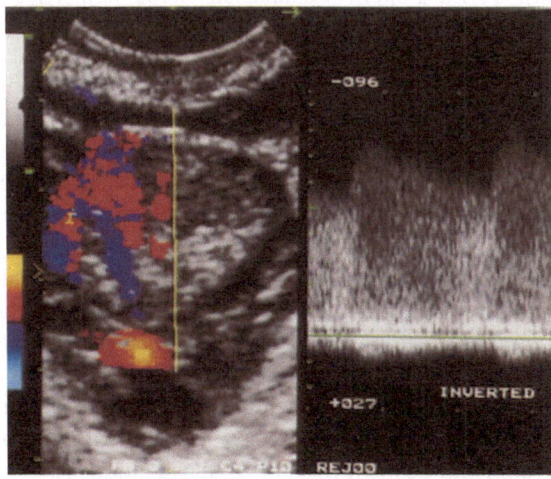

Fig. 3. Colour Doppler scan shows increased vascularity in a solid adnexal mass, which represents tubal pregnancy

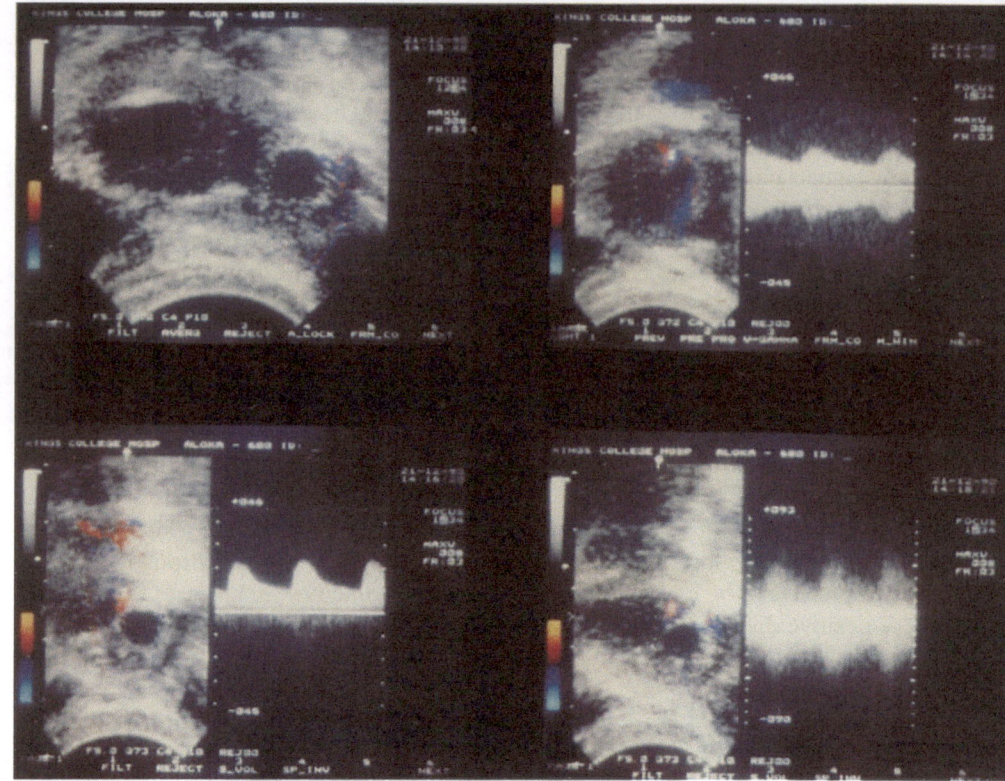

Fig. 4. Technique of Doppler examination in a case of ectopic pregnancy. B-mode scan (*upper left*) shows the right ovary and a small empty sac-like area adjacent to it, which may represent a bulging corpus luteum or an ectopic pregnancy. Colour Doppler examination of the ovary (*upper right*) confirms the presence of the corpus luteum by demonstrating its typical blood supply. Blood vessels which are supplying the adjacent sac are visualized separately (*lower left* and *right*). Pulsed Doppler examination shows flow velocity waveforms typical of peritrophoblastic flow

pregnancy actually have a miscarriage, the impact of improved diagnostic accuracy in terms of reducing the patients' anxiety and need for further investigation is greater than in patients with proven ectopic pregnancies. By using colour Doppler it is also possible to prevent the diagnosis of early intra-uterine pregnancies in patients with a pseudogestational sac. The absence of peritrophoblastic flow helps to avoid this common cause of diagnostic uncertainty.

Colour Doppler studies of blood flow in ectopic pregnancy increase the accuracy of ultrasound diagnosis of this condition. The detection of characteristic blood flow allows a definite diagnosis of ectopic pregnancy to be made in patients with non-specific adnexal masses on the B-mode scan. It may also help to avoid a false-positive diagnosis of ectopic pregnancy in patients with a bulging corpus luteum or in women with other forms of tubal pathology. In cases with absent adnexal pathology, a corpus luteum may be identified and used as a guide to search

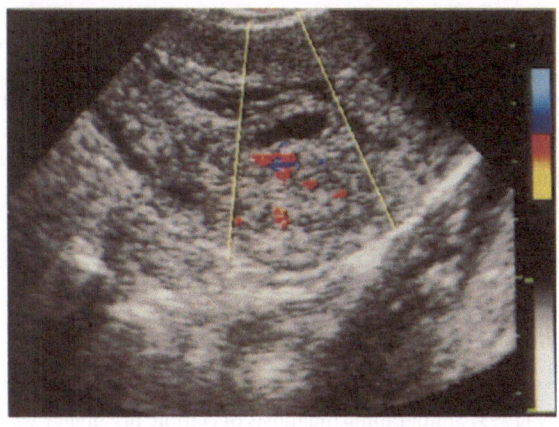

Fig. 5. The presence of peritrophoblastic flow in a case of an empty intra-uterine sac helps to distinguish it from a pseudogestational sac

for an ectopic pregnancy. It remains to be established whether an apparent decrease in the vascular supply to an ectopic sac indicates poor viability and hence the selection of patients who may benefit from conservative, non-interventional management. Furthermore, colour Doppler findings enable a confident diagnosis of failed intra-uterine pregnancy, even in patients with no visible intra-uterine sac, and enable accurate distinction between pseudogestational sac and early intra-uterine pregnancy.

References

1. Barnea ER, Oelsner G, Benveniste R, Romero R, DeCherney AH (1986) Progesterone, estradiol, and alpha human chorionic gonadotropin secretion in patients with ectopic pregnancy. J Clin Endocrinol Metab 62: 529
2. Bourne TH, Jurkovic D, Waterstone J, Campbell S, Collins WP (1991) Intra-follicular blood flow during human ovulation. Ultrasound Obstet Gynecol 1: 53
3. Burden HB (1972) Adrenergic innervation in ovaries of the rat and guinea pig. Am J Anat 133: 455
4. Cacciatore B, Stenman UH, Ylostalo P (1989) Comparison of abdominal and vaginal sonography in suspected ectopic pregnancy. Obstet Gynecol 73: 770
5. Cacciatore B, Ulf-Hakan S, Ylostalo P (1990) Diagnosis of ectopic pregnancy by vaginal ultrasonography in combination with a discriminatory serum hCG level of 1000 IU/l (IRP). Br J Obstet Gynaecol 97: 904–908
6. Collins PW, Jurkovic D, Bourne TH, Kurjak A, Campbell S (1991) Ovarian morphology, endocrine function and intra-follicular blood flow during the peri-ovulatory period. Hum Reprod 6: 319
7. Devroey P, Camus M, Palermo G, Smitz J, Van Waesberghe L, Wisanto A, Wijbo I, Van Steirteghem AC (1990) Placental production of estradiol and progresterone after oocyte donation in patients with primary ovarian failure. Am J Obstet Gynecol 162: 66
8. Emerson DS, Cartier MS, Altieri LA et al (1992) Diagnostic efficacy of endovaginal color Doppler flow imaging in an ectopic pregnancy screening program. Radiology 183: 413–420
9. Hubinont CJ, Thomas C, Schwers JF (1987) Luteal function in ectopic pregnancy. Am J Obstet Gynecol 156: 669

10. Jurkovic D, Jauniaux E, Kurjak A, Hustin J, Campbell S, Nicolaides KH (1991) Transvaginal color Doppler assessment of the uteroplacental circulation in early pregancy. Obstet Gynecol 77: 365
11. Jurkovic D, Bourne TH, Jauniaux E, Campbell S, Collins WP (1992) Transvaginal color Doppler study of blood flow in ectopic pregnancies. Fertil Steril 57: 68
12. Kirchler HC, Kolle D, Schwegel P (1992) Changes in tubal blood flow in evaluating ectopic pregnancy. Ultrasound Obstet Gynecol 2: 283
13. Kurjak A, Zalud I, Jurkovic D, Alfirevic Z, Miljan M (1989) Transvaginal color Doppler for the assessment of pelvic circulation. Acta obstet Gynecol Scand 68: 131
14. Kurjak A, Zalud I, Schulman (1991) Ectopic pregnancy: transvaginal color Doppler identifies trophoblastic flow in suspicious adnexa. J Clin Ultrasound 10: 685
15. Pellierito JS, Taylor KJW, Quadens-Case C, et al (1992) Ectopic pregnancy: evaluation with endovaginal color flow imaging. Radiology 183: 407
16. Randall S, Buckley H, Fox H (1987) Placentation in the fallopian tube. Int J Gynecol Pathol 6: 132
17. Russel SA, Filly RA, Damato N (1993) Sonographic diagnosis of ectopic pregnancy with endovaginal probes: What has really changed. J Ultrasound Med 3: 145
18. Schulman H, Fleischer A, Farmakides G, Bracero L, Rochelson B, Grunfeld L (1986) Development of uterine artery compliance in pregnancy as detected by Doppler ultrasound. Am J Obstet Gynecol 155: 1031
19. Shapiro BS, Cullen M, Taylor KJW, DeCherney AH (1988) Transvaginal ultrasonography for the diagnosis of ectopic pregnancy. Fertil Steril 50: 425
20. Steer CV, Campbell S, Pampiglione JS, Kingsland CR, Mason BA, Collins WP (1990) Transvaginal colour flow imaging of the uterine arteries during the ovarian and menstrual cycles. Hum Reprod 5: 391
21. Stiller RJ, Haynes de Regt R, Blair E (1989) Transvaginal ultrasonography in patients at risk for ectopic pregnancy. Am J Obstet Gynecol 161: 930
22. Taylor KJW, Ramos IM, Feyock AL, et al (1989) Ectopic pregnancy: duplex Doppler evaluation. Radiology 173: 93
23. Tekay A, Jouppila P (1992) Color Doppler flow as an indicator of trophoblastic activity in tubal pregnancies detected by transvaginal ultrasound. Obstet Gynecol 80: 995
24. Timor-Tritch IE, Yeh MN, Peisner DB, Lesser KB, Slavik TA (1989) The use of transvaginal sonography in the diagnosis of ectopic pregnancy. Am J Obstet Gynecol 161: 157
25. Wiltbank MC, Gallagher KP, Dysko R, Keyes PL (1989) Regulation of blood flow to the rabbit corpus luteum: effects of estradiol and human chorionic gonadotropin. Endocrinology 124: 605

Hystero-Contrast-Salpingography – Colour Doppler and the Study of Fallopian Tube Patency

T.H. Bourne and E. Hacket

Introduction

Approximately 10% of couples in the United Kingdom will be destined to suffer from infertility, which can be defined as a failure to conceive after regular sexual intercourse for a period of 1 year. The investigation of such couples amounts to a major investment both in time and money. Prominent amongst these investigations is the assessment of fallopian tube patency. The reasons for this are threefold:

1. To diagnose a cause of infertility.
2. If at least one tube is patent, it might be possible to stimulate folliculogenesis.
3. If both tubes are blocked, the couple can be referred for in vitro fertilisation (IVF).

The amount of information that is required about tubal patency in order to effectively manage a patient is uncertain. Many would say that far more subtle details of structure and function are required than simply whether a tube is blocked or not. However, it can be argued that this may be all that is required to decide on a reasonable treatment strategy for the patient. In the event of tubal damage, surgery may be considered, although the outcome is not good following such procedures. Unless adhesions are minimal, the likely pregnancy rate following surgery is of the order of 40% or less and the subsequent ectopic pregnancy rate is significant. In contrast, the data of Tan et al. [12] suggest the cumulative pregnancy rate after three cycles of IVF may be as high as 60%, although it must be appreciated that this rate applies to younger women and tends to decline with age. Subjecting women to tubal surgery in some cases may merely lead to delayed treatment by IVF, which in turn will both decrease the likely "take home" baby rate and increase the cost of the procedure [7]. What is needed is a simple out-patient test that will select those women with bilaterally blocked tubes in order that they can be referred at an early stage for IVF. Candidates for this test are laparoscopy, hystero-salpingography (HSG) and hystero-contrast-salpingography (hycosy).

Laparoscopy is an invasive procedure that in most cases requires a general anaesthetic. It provides useful information regarding the presence or absence of both endometriosis and adhesions, but tells us nothing about the internal structure of the uterus and ovaries. HSG is less invasive, but involves exposure to radiation and demands the services of a radiology department.

The use of ultrasound in this context offers distinct advantages. B-mode imaging alone provides information about ovarian morphology and volume, congenital and acquired uterine abnormalities and, with colour Doppler, may also give an indication of function [2, 11]. Hycosy uses non-iodinated contrast agents and so allergies are less likely; it can be performed in the out-patient clinic or office and appears to provide similar information regarding tubal patency as laparoscopy and HSG. We can now consider this technique in more detail.

Procedure

Practical Aspects

The examination of the pre-menopausal uterus, tubes and ovaries has been described [3]. However, it is with the use of contrast material that hycosy differs from the normal transvaginal ultrasound examination. Our experience has been with sterile saline and a suspension of gas microbubbles stabilised on galactose microparticles ("Echovist", Schering AG, Berlin). The procedure can be carried out in any gynaecology clinic that is equipped with ultrasound equipment, and it is no more invasive than the insertion of an intra-uterine contraceptive device. As with any technique involving instrumentation of the cervix, resuscitation facilities must be available to deal with possible vagal reactions. Contra-indications include galactosaemia (when using Echovist as the contrast agent), concurrent acute genital infections, pregnancy and heavy vaginal bleeding. Hycosy should be carried out in the first half of the menstrual cycle to reduce the chances of disturbing an early pregnancy, as well as any risk of pelvic infection.

Having passed a Cusco's speculum and disinfected the vagina, a 2-mm uterine catheter is inserted into the uterine cavity. As the initial part of the examination involves examining the endometrium, better results may be obtained by inserting the catheter only as far as the internal os. The catheter balloon must not be fully inflated in the cervical canal, as this will cause discomfort, but some degree of inflation will prevent excessive backflow of contrast. Examination of the uterine cavity is better performed using sterile saline rather than an hyperechoic contrast medium such as Echovist [1]. Very clear images of endometrial pathology can be obtained by injecting saline into the cavity [4], whilst the strong acoustic shadow cast by media such as Echovist will often obscure details of endometrial morphology (Fig. 1). It may be necessary to inject up to 15 ml of sterile saline to obtain optimal views of the cavity. The diagnostic accuracy of transvaginal ultrasonography compared to hysteroscopy has been shown to be similar. In a study of 200 patients, assuming hysteroscopy to be the gold standard, the sensitivity of transvaginal ultrasonography for the detection of uterine abnormalities was 98.9% and the false-positive rate 5.5% [8]. The addition of intracavity saline enhances the diagnostic potential of ultrasound further, particularly for the assessment of polyps (Fig. 2).

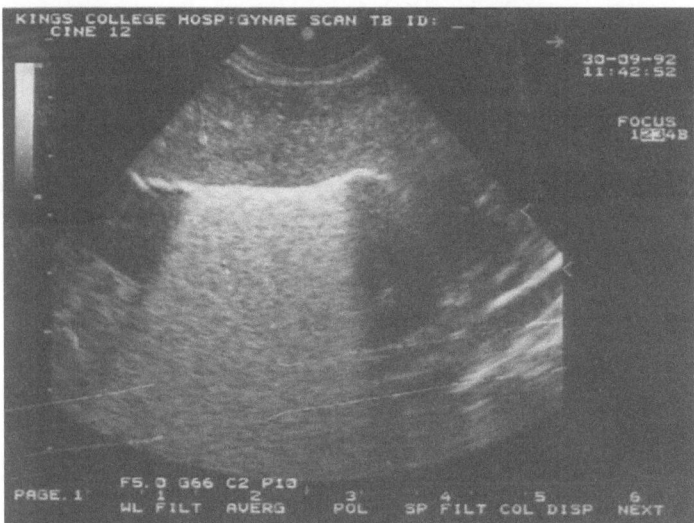

Fig. 1. Ultrasound contrast (Echovist) has been introduced into the uterine cavity. Note the strong acoustic shadow. It is not possible to visualise details of the posterior wall of the endometrial cavity or uterine wall

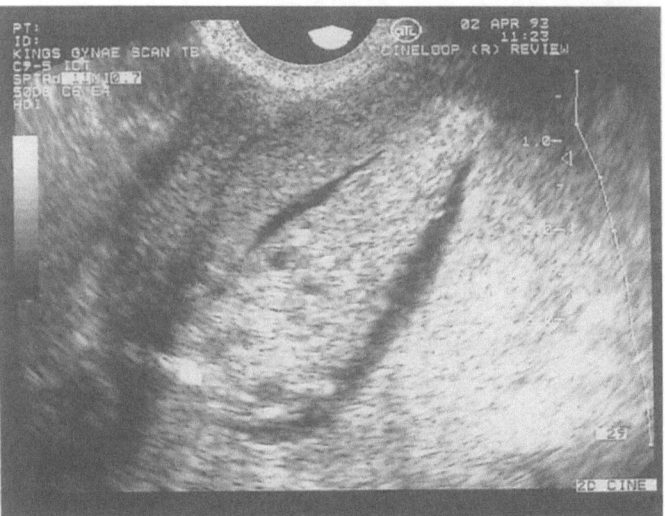

Fig. 2. Longitudinal view of the uterus. A total of 10 ml sterile saline has been injected into the cavity, and a large endometrial polyp can be seen floating free of the cavity. This patient had been taking 20 mg tamoxifen over a period of 12 months. Subsequent histology of the polyp revealed a focus of atypical hyperplasia (from [4] courtesy of the International Society for Ultrasound in Obstetrics and Gynecology)

Having assessed the uterus, the catheter can be pushed fully into the endo-metrial cavity, and the balloon fully inflated. Again care must be taken at this time, as the amount of patient discomfort associated with the procedure seems related mostly to fully inflating the uterine catheter in the cervical canal or to injecting too great a volume of contrast too quickly. In the case of Echovist, the contrast agent consists of galactose monosaccharide microparticles (50% < 2 μ) in a 20% (wt/vol) solution of galactose [9] (Fig. 3). The suspension is prepared immediately before

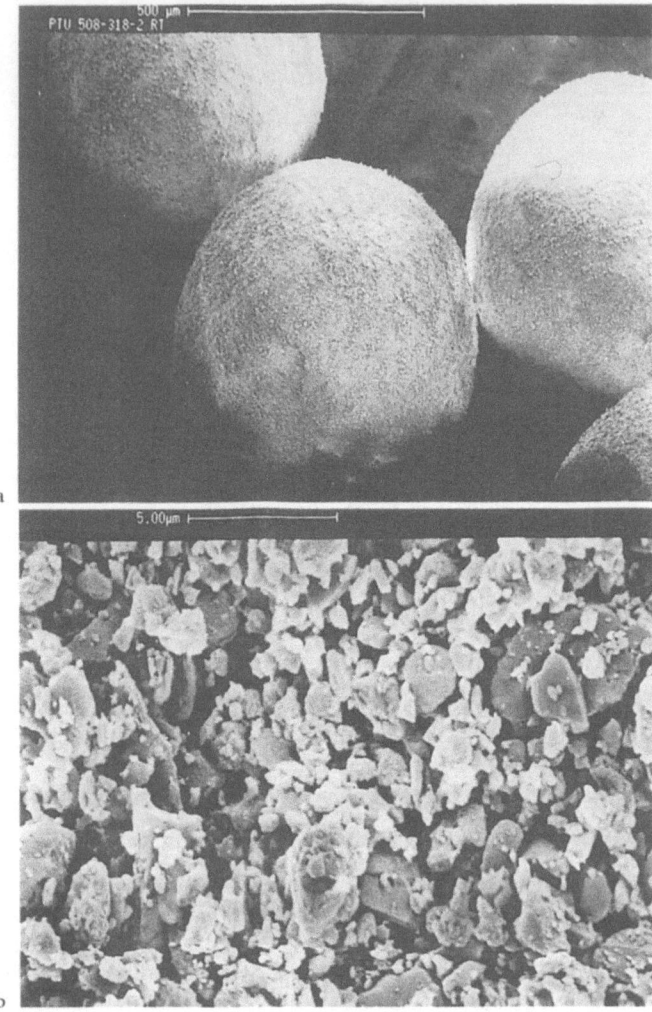

Fig. 3a,b. Micrographs of granule/microparticles of a galactose-based echocontrast agent. **a** Galactose granule at ×80. **b** Surface detail of a granule at ×5000 showing the microparticles that form the granules. Air microbubbles are trapped and stabilised in the spaces around the microparticles. (Figure courtesy of Dr. R. Schlief, Schering AG, Berlin)

injection. Having filled the uterine cavity with a few milliliters of contrast media, the tubes should then begin to fill quickly. In the majority of cases B-mode imaging alone will be sufficient to visualise flow of contrast through the tube (Figs. 4, 5), with spill into the peritoneal cavity diagnostic of patency. The flow in the tube should change easily with the degree of pressure on the syringe. Tubal patency can otherwise be defined as the visualisation of steady tubal flow lasting at least 10 s in

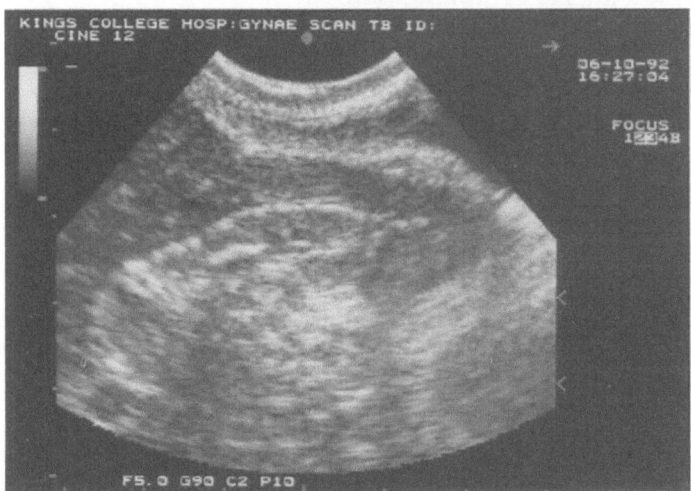

Fig. 4. In this unusual view, the fallopian tube can be seen clearly just before the injection of ultrasound contrast (see Fig. 5)

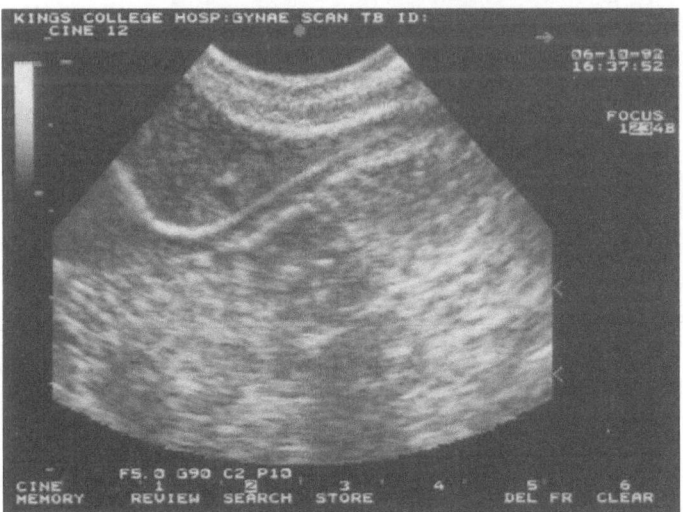

Fig. 5. Contrast (Echovist) can be clearly seen filling the fallopian tube in B-mode imaging. Colour Doppler is not necessary in this case to make the diagnosis of patency

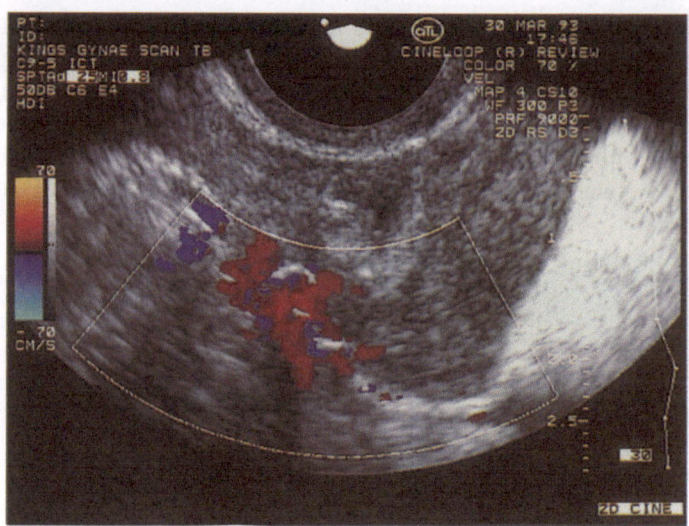

Fig. 6. The diagnosis of patency has already been made using B-mode imaging; however, the colour Doppler gate has been positioned over the tube to illustrate the presence of flow in the tube

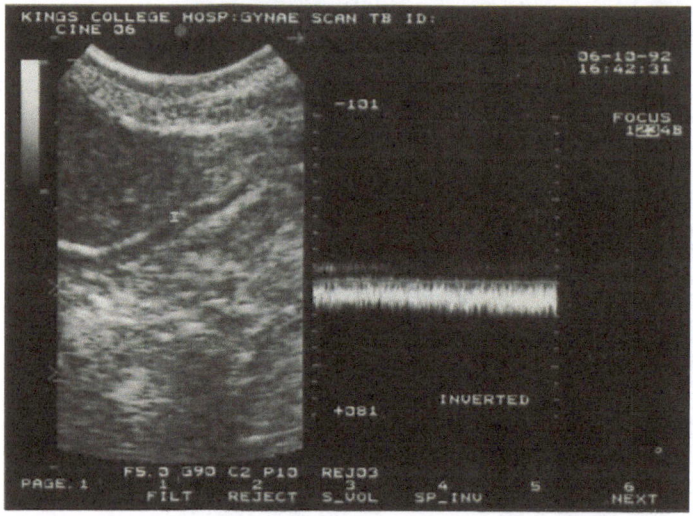

Fig. 7. A pulsed Doppler range gate has been placed over the tube; a pulsed Doppler waveform typical of tubal patency is shown

one imaged tubal section. Typically, 10 ml contrast media injected in 1- to 2-ml aliquots will be needed up to a total maximum possible volume of 30 ml.

In some patients it will not be possible to visualise the entire tube, the result possibly being a false-positive diagnosis of tubal blockage. It is in the relatively small, but important number of patients in which this problem arises that Doppler has a role to play. The colour Doppler gate can be placed over the presumed mural portion of the tube and will detect the movement of contrast (Fig. 6). This can be used to direct the positioning of a pulsed Doppler range gate to obtain a flow velocity waveform. The demonstration of a pulsed Doppler waveform from the tube is diagnostic of tubal patency; the amplitude of the waveform will be proportional to the amount of pressure put on the syringe (Fig. 7).

Comparison of Hystero-Contrast-Salpingography with Hystero-Salpingography and Laparoscopy

Any consideration of the efficacy of hycosy for the study of tubal patency is complicated by the fact that the reference methods of HSG and laparoscopy themselves have limitations. Despite this, they are used as "gold standard" reference procedures against which hycosy must compare favourably to find a clinically useful role. However, it should be remembered that limited concordance has been reported between laparoscopy and HSG, whilst there is little information to assess the inter-observer error in the assessment of tubal patency using either reference method. Initial reports investigating the use of hycosy and conventional methods of assessing tubal patency have been promising. In their initial report, Schlief and Deichart [10] found that hycosy detected 47% of blocked tubes with a false-positive rate of 14.8% when using B-mode imaging alone (Table 1). However, in the small number of cases when they used colour Doppler, they detected all the blocked tubes, whilst reducing the false-positive rate to 4.0% (Table 2). These data are similar to our small experience at King's College Hospital (Table 3), where again all the blocked tubes were recognised, with a false-positive rate of just 10.5%. It is likely that the slightly higher false-positive rate in our hands reflected the

Table 1. Comparison of hystero-contrast-salpingography (Hycosy; B-mode ultrasonography) and hystero-salpingography (HSG) or laparoscopy

		Hycosy		All
		+	−	
Tubal Blockage				
(one or both)	+	7	8	15
	−	0	54	54
	All	7	62	69

Prevalence of blocked tubes: $(15/54) \times 100 = 27.8\%$.
Detection rate: $(7/15) \times 100 = 46.7\%$.
False-positive rate: $8/54 = 14.8\%$.
Positive predictive value: $(7/7) \times 100 = 100\%$.
Calculated from data in [10].

Table 2. Comparison of hystero-contrast-salpingography (Hycosy) with Doppler (Duplex or colour) and hystero-salpingography (HSG) or laparoscopy

		Hycosy		All
		+	−	
Tubal Blockage				
(both)	+	2	0	2
	−	2	23	25
	All	4	23	27

Prevalence of blocked tubes: $(2/27) \times 100 = 7.4\%$.
Detection rate: $(2/2) \times 100 = 100.0\%$.
False-positive rate: $(2/25) \times 100 = 4.0\%$.
Positive predictive value: $(2/4) \times 100 = 50.0\%$.
Calculated from data in [10].

Table 3. Comparison of hystero-contrast-salpingography (Hycosy) with colour Doppler and hystero-salpingography (HSG)

		Hycosy		All
		+	−	
Tubal Blockage				
(both)	+	4	0	4
	−	2[a]	17[b]	19
	All	6	17	23

Prevalence of blocked tubes: $(4/23) \times 100 = 17.3\%$.
Detection rate: $(4/4) \times 100 = 100.0\%$.
False-positive rate: $(2/19) \times 100 = 10.5\%$.
Positive predictive value: $(4/6) \times 100 = 66.7\%$.
[a] One tube patent by HSG.
[b] Four unilateral tubes by both HSG and Hycosy; one unilateral tube by Hycosy alone.

learning curve associated with the procedure. The information currently available suggests that colour Doppler adds significantly to overall test performance. In particular, tubes thought to be blocked on B-mode imaging can be seen to be patent by the demonstration of contrast flow using Doppler. In a more recent publication, Degenhardt et al. [6] demonstrated that the findings using hycosy were similar to HSG and laparoscopy in between 92% and 95% of the 61 women studied. Surprisingly, most of these examinations were carried out without the aid of Doppler. It is of interest in this study that a linear score to assess patient discomfort was included: 22% of patients had no pain during the procedure, 75% little pain, with only 2.4% complaining of severe pain. In contrast, the data of Balen et al. [1] based on 25 patients are less favourable. In their series complete agreement between hycosy and HSG or laparoscopy occurred in only 54% of cases.

One of the largest studies evaluating hycosy is as yet unpublished and consists of the data from the open clinical phase IIIb study of the use of Echovist (data on file at Schering Health Care Ltd., 1994). A total of 311 women were recruited to this multicentre trial. In all cases hycosy was performed on an out-patient basis with the aid of Doppler when required, and only 11% of women received any sort of premedication. The results from this study suggest a high level of agreement between hycosy and reference procedures for the diagnosis of tubal patency. The detection rate for patency was 87% compared to HSG and 95.5% compared to laparoscopy. The false-positive rate was less than 12% in comparison to HSG and 26% with laparoscopy. In 65% of cases, hycosy offered additional diagnostic information not available from the reference method. This reflects the advantages of ultrasound discussed earlier in this text. This study is informative, as it highlights some of the problems that may be encountered with the procedure. A total of 15% of women reported some sort of reaction. The most common complaints were nausea, faintness and flushing. The design of this trial makes it difficult to derive a clear picture of the degree of discomfort associated with hycosy. However, only 22% of the women had pain that was felt to require any therapy, most of which was in the form of simple oral analgesics. Our experience was that pain is usually related to inflation of the uterine catheter balloon when incorrectly placed or too rapid an injection of contrast into the uterus, resulting in tubal spasm. Discomfort at the time of the procedure was often associated with tubal block. Invariably our patients, when asked, found hycosy less painful than HSG.

Future Prospects

It is important to remember that, as with any practical procedure, there is a learning curve. The consensus view is that about 20 hycosy examinations are needed in order to obtain good results. The data from the multicentre trial above must be looked at in this context, with experience the performance of hycosy may improve further. Whilst it seems apparent that hycosy gives similar data to other reference methods regarding the presence or absence of tubal patency, there are limitations. Hycosy gives little information about fimbrial adhesions; furthermore, the exact location of tubal block is difficult to ascertain using this technique. This must be balanced against the increased diagnostic information associated with the use of ultrasound, which by its nature is able to look inside structures and not just at them. The use of Doppler in the procedure is one of the few clear indications for its use in gynaecological practice; it can be utilised to enhance the recognition of patent tubes and thus reduce the number of tubes falsely reported as being blocked (Fig. 8). It is clear that transvaginal ultrasonography is already an accurate test for the detection of uterine pathology. The addition of a negative contrast agent serves to enhance this ability, particularly for the recognition of polyps. In this context, positive contrast agents such as Echovist may in fact make the assessment of the

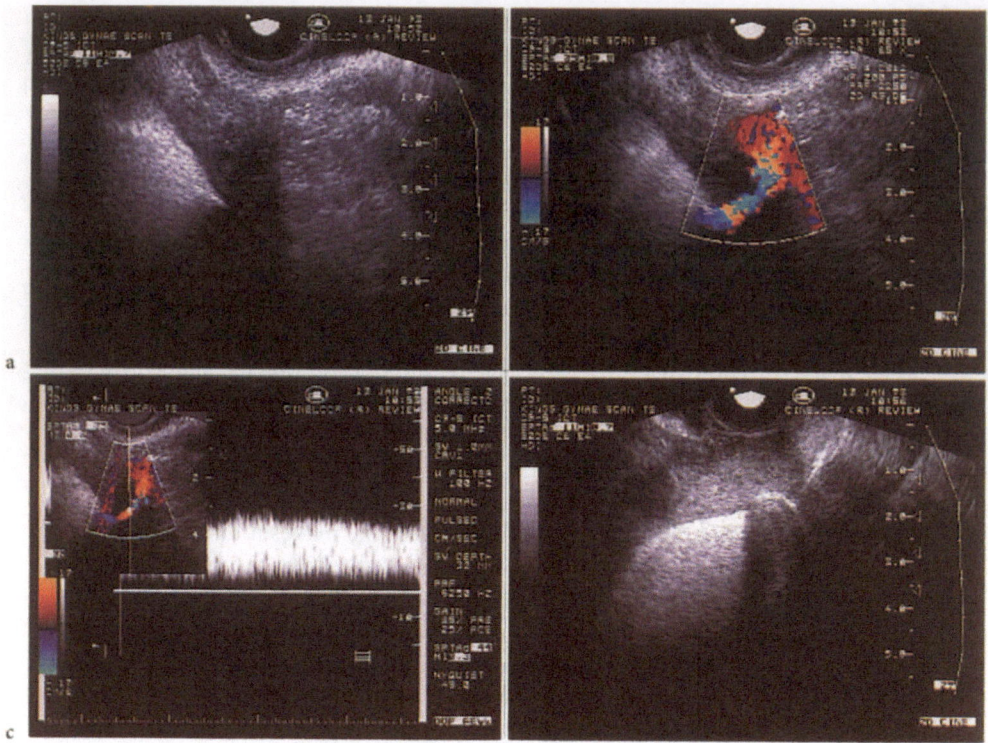

Fig. 8. a,b In this series of images, colour Doppler has been used to locate an area of flow in the tube not visible using B-mode imaging alone; **c** a pulsed Doppler range gate use to produce a characteristic flow velocity waveform consistent with tubal patency; **d** further example of tubal filling with contrast medium using B-mode imaging

uterus more difficult, their use being mainly applicable to the diagnosis of fallopian tube patency.

Finally, it is necessary to ask what the potential place of hycosy is in the infertility work-up. It is likely that it will serve as a screening test to select infertile women for appropriate further investigation. If it is found that a women has at least one patent tube using hycosy, she could be entered for follicular stimulation without recourse to further tubal investigation. If the tubes are blocked, HSG could then be used as a second-stage test to check the location of the block, with laparoscopy reserved if the occlusion is felt to be fimbrial in origin.

Certainly it is our belief that transvaginal ultrasonography should be an integral part of the investigation of infertile women. Details of both ovarian and uterine morphology as well as blood flow can be obtained. The advent of ultrasound contrast now means that an assessment of tubal patency can be made at the same time. Given the relatively poor outcome of surgery for tubal occlusion, a more radical role for hycosy might be envisaged. Hycosy could be performed at the first visit for the investigation of infertility. Those with bilateral tubal block may be sent directly for IVF with only minimal further investigation (assuming that the partner is not azospermic), whilst those with patent tubes may be offered follicular stimulation.

Larger studies will be needed to define the precise place of this test in the investigation of the infertile couple as well as its cost implications. However, in an increasingly cost-conscious health environment, the introduction of a simple, efficient out-patient test such as this must have its attractions. Furthermore, as with many other areas involving ultrasound, the problems of quality control and training will have to be grasped. Many of these issues have been reviewed elsewhere [5].

Acknowledgements. We would like to thank Keymed (Southend-on-sea, Essex, UK) and the Aloka Company Ltd. (Tokyo, Japan) for the use of their ultrasound equipment. We are grateful to Schering Health Care Ltd. for their support of the gynaecological ultrasound clinic.

References

1. Balen FG, Allen CM, Siddle NC, Lees WR (1993) Ultrasound contrast hystero-salpingography–evaluation as an outpatient procedure. Br J Radiol 66: 592–599
2. Bourne TH, Jurkovic D, Waterstone J, Campbell S, Collins WP (1991) Intrafollicular blood flow during human ovulation. Ultrasound Obstet Gynecol 1: 53–59
3. Bourne TH (1991) Transvaginal color Doppler in gynecology. Ultrasound Obstet Gynecol 1: 359–373
4. Bourne TH, Lawton F, Leather A, Granberg S, Campbell S, Collins WP (1994) Use of intracavity saline instillation and transvaginal ultrasonography to detect tamoxifen-associated endometrial polyps. Ultrasound Obstets Gynecol 4: 73–75
5. Campbell S, Bourne TH, Tan SL (1994) Hysterosalpingo contrast sonography (HyCoSy) and its future role within the investigation of infertility in Europe. Ultrasound Obstets Gynecol 4: 245–253
6. Degenhardt F, Jibril S, Eisenhauer B, Gohde M, Schlosser HW (1993) Vaginal hysterosalpingo-contrast-sonography. BMUS Bull Nov: 36 37
7. Granberg M (1993) Is IVF really expensive? Lakareesallskapet, Handleingar Hygiea, OB32 P
8. Narayan R, Goswamy R (1993) Transvaginal sonography of the uterine cavity with hysteroscopic correlation in the investigation of infertility. Ultrasound Obstets Gynecol 3: 129–133
9. Schlief R (1987) First steps in ultrasound contrast media. In: Felix R (ed) Contrast media from the past to the future. Thieme, Stuttgart, pp 179–187
10. Schlief R, Deichart U (1991) Hysterosalpingo-contrast sonography of the uterus and fallopian tubes: results of a clinical trial of a new contrast medium in 120 patients. Radiology 178: 213–215
11. Steer CV, Campbell S, Pampiglione J, Kingsland C, Mason BA, Collins WP (1990) Transvaginal color flow imaging of the uterine arteries during the ovarian and menstrual cycles. Hum Reprod 5: 391–395
12. Tan SL, Steer C, Royston P, Rizk P, Mason BA, Campbell S (1990) Conception rates and in vitro fertilisation. Lancet 335: 229

IV.   Embryo or Fetus

Assessment of the Early Foetal Circulation

J.W. WLADIMIROFF and I.P. VAN SPLUNDER

Introduction

With the advent of transvaginal Doppler ultrasound, it became feasible to examine the maternal uterine and foetal circulation as early as the first trimester of pregnancy. Particularly during the late first and early second trimester, marked developmental changes occur both at foetal and placental level which should have an impact on foetal cardiovascular performance. Foetal heart rate changes from 170–180 bpm to 140–150 bpm with appearance of beat to beat variation most likely resulting from parasympathetic nerve development [20]. At the same time there is a remarkable differentiation in foetal movement patterns. Furthermore, around 14 weeks a continuous intervillous flow pattern has been observed [11]. This is associated with an abrupt increase of the mean uterine blood flow velocity, which possibly corresponds to the complete dislocation of the trophoblast plugs, allowing uninhibited blood supply to the intervillous space. An overview on human foetal cardiovascular Doppler research in early pregnancy will be presented.

The transvaginal technique will result in a closer approach of the foetus and therefore allow higher carrier frequencies and thus higher image resolution. Doppler waveform recording may be attempted following visualization of foetal cardiac or extra-cardiac vessel structures. Colour-coded Doppler will be helpful in locating arterial blood flow, as well as intra-cardiac and venous blood flow in early pregnancy (Figs. 1, 2). When applying Doppler techniques, energy levels should be taken into account. In early pregnancy Doppler studies, spatial peak temporal average (SPTA) levels below 100 mW/cm² were aimed for (See pp. 88–98).

Whereas under 13–14 weeks of gestation the superiority of the transvaginal approach is unchallenged, the growing foetus will render this technique increasingly difficult beyond that stage of pregnancy. Beyond 14 weeks foetal flow velocity waveforms will nearly always be obtained by means of transabdominal Doppler ultrasound.

Extra-cardiac Arterial Flow Velocity Waveforms

Waveforms have so far been studied in the umbilical artery [2, 3, 6, 14, 21, 23], descending aorta [14, 21, 23] and intracerebral arteries [15, 22]. Intracerebral waveforms can be obtained from the internal carotid or middle cerebral artery

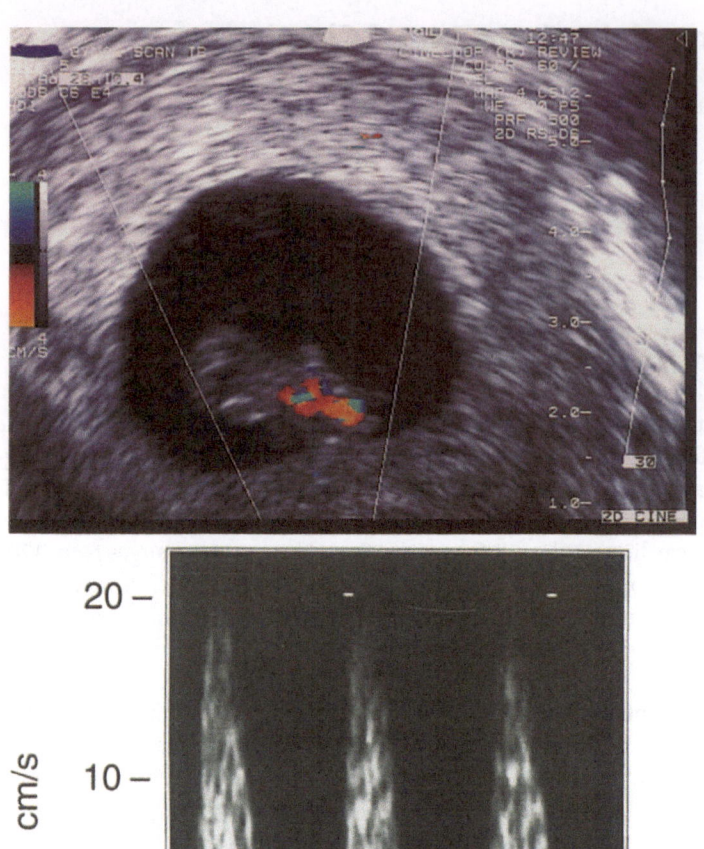

Fig. 1a,b. Colour-coded Doppler image of the foetal circulation at 8½ weeks of gestation. *Red* represents the descending aorta

[23]. Distinction between these two vessels is often not possible. Before 10 weeks of gestation, all waveforms depict absent end-diastolic flow velocities, suggesting a high vascular resistance at foetal and umbilical placental level compared with late pregnancy [3].

Figures 1 and 2 represent a waveform recording from the descending aorta and the umbilical artery and vein at 8 weeks of gestation. Note the pulsatile nature of umbilical venous blood flow during this early stage of pregnancy.

Wladimiroff et al. established the appearance of end-diastolic flow velocities in over 50% of intracerebral artery flow velocity waveforms between 10 and 12 weeks of gestation, whereas in the umbilical artery and descending aorta end-

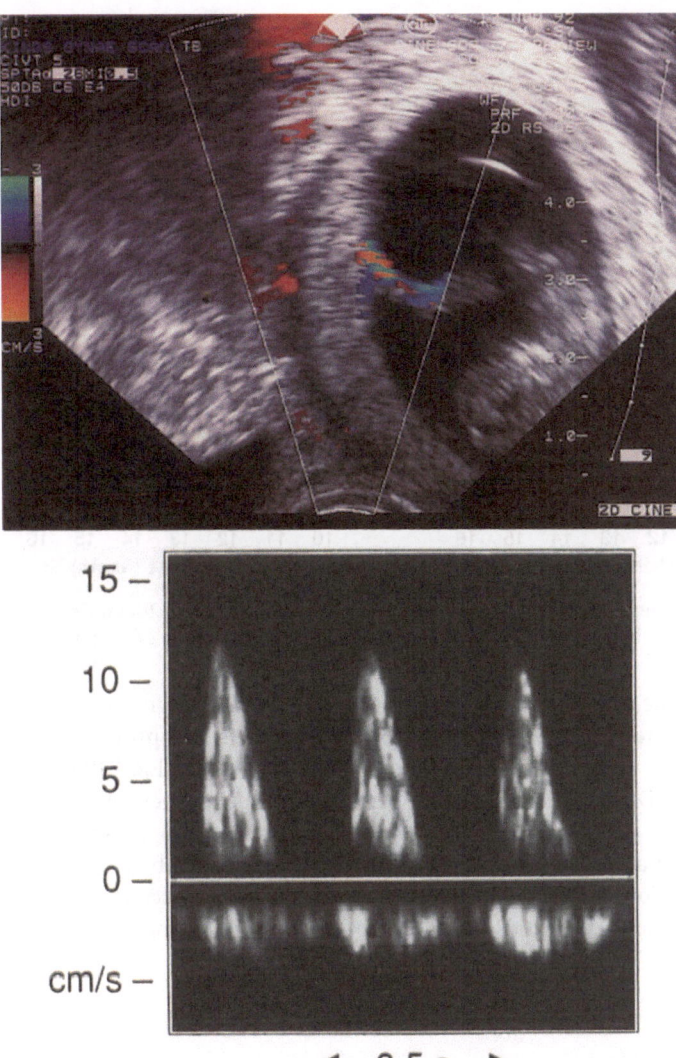

Fig. 2a,b. Colour imaging (**a**) and flow velocity waveforms (**b**) in the umbilical artery and vein. Note the absence of end-diastolic flow velocities in the umbilical artery and the pulsatile nature of umbilical venous blood flow

diastolic velocities are still absent [23]. These data suggest a relatively low cerebral vascular resistance and as a result preferential blood flow to the brain under otherwise physiological circumstances. However, after 12 weeks end-diastolic velocities also gradually appear in the umbilical artery and descending aorta, indicating a reduction in foetal placental vascular resistance [23].

Reduction in vascular resistance was also reported for the uterine artery in this early stage of pregnancy [3, 10]. Of interest at this point is the secundary tropho-

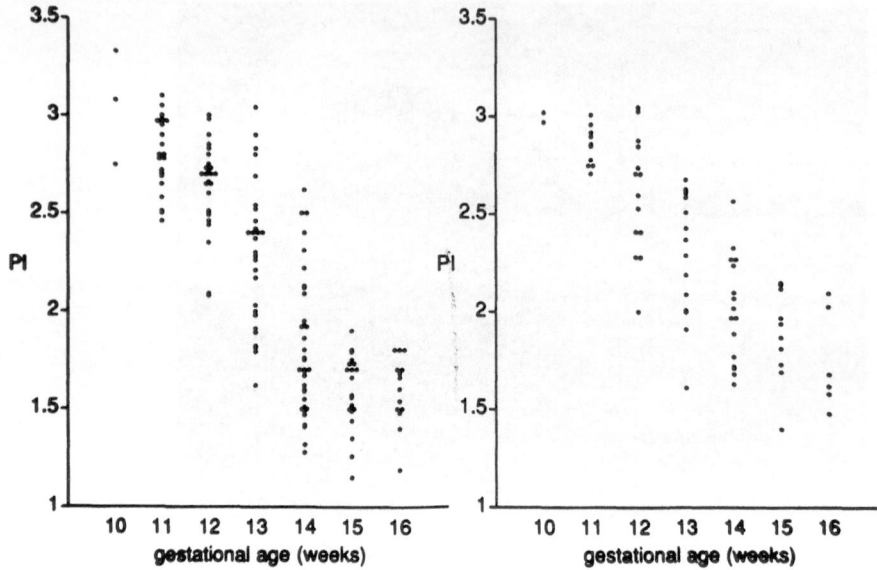

Fig. 3. Pulsatility index (*PI*) in the umbilical artery (*left*; $n = 152$) and foetal descending aorta (*right*; $n = 74$) relative to gestational age between 11 and 16 weeks of gestation

blast invasion of the spiral arteries in early second trimester pregnancy, resulting in low-resistance utero-placental vessels [15]. This will ensure optimal placental perfusion, which is necessary to accommodate the increased blood flow to the developing foetus. During the early second trimester of pregnancy, end-diastolic flow velocities will be consistently present in all three aforementioned foetal arterial vessels and a drop in pulsatility index (PI) has been established. Figure 3 displays the reduction in PI in the umbilical artery and foetal descending aorta as a result of the appearance of end-diastolic velocities in these vessels.

Intra-cardiac Flow Velocity Waveforms

Transvaginal foetal echocardiography has been shown to be effective in the visualization of normal early foetal cardiac anatomy and, therefore, suggested to have a significant potential for the diagnosis of gross foetal cardiac anomalies during the late first and early second trimester of pregnancy [4]. Doppler flow velocities have been collected at atrio-ventricular and outflow tract level [22].

Transtricuspid and transmitral waveforms can be obtained from the two-dimensional image in the four-chamber view. The sample volume (0.1–0.3 cm) should be placed immediately distal to the tricuspid and mitral valve. The interrogation angle should always be kept at 20° or less.

Figure 4 depicts an atrio-ventricular waveform recording at 10 weeks, consisting of the early diastolic or E-wave component and late diastolic or A-wave component and demonstrating that differentiation between passive diastolic filling and

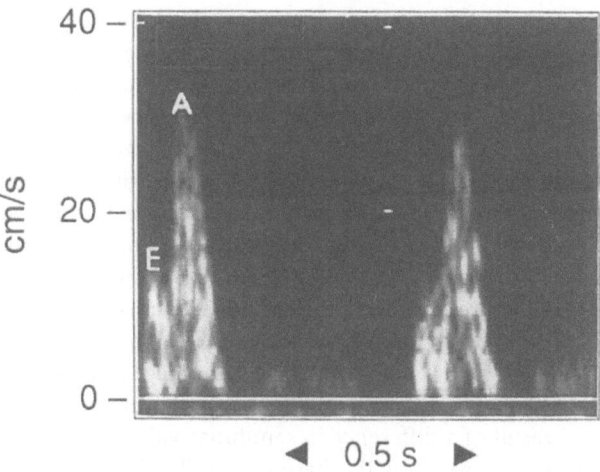

Fig. 4. Waveform recording at the level of the foetal atrio-ventricular valves at 10 weeks, depicting the E-wave (early diastolic filling) and the
A-wave (atrial contraction)

atrial contraction is feasible as early as this. Of interest is the relatively low peak E-wave velocity when compared with peak A-wave velocity, resulting in an E to A ratio of approximately 0.5 as opposed to E to A ratios ranging between 0.8 and 0.9 in late pregnancy [19, 22]. The clear A-wave dominance at the atrio-ventricular level reflects the relative stiffness of the cardiac ventricles in early gestation. At 11–12 weeks, mean peak E-wave and A-wave velocities of 20.5 ± 3.2 cm/s and 38.6 ± 4.7 cm/s have been established [22]. Both at mitral and tricuspid valve level there is a marked rise in peak E-wave velocities and E to A ratios with advancing gestational age. This suggests a shift of blood flow from late towards early diastole, which may be due to increased ventricular compliance and/or raised ventricular relaxation rate [25].

After 12 weeks transtricuspid time-averaged, peak E-wave and peak A-wave velocities are higher than transmitral flow velocities [25]. Since volume flow is equal to time-averaged velocity multiplied by vessel area, the higher transtricuspid time-averaged velocities may reflect increased right ventricular stroke volume and output.

At outflow tract level, aortic and pulmonary artery flow velocities may also be recorded as early as 10–11 weeks of gestation. Velocity waveforms in the ascending aorta are obtained from the five-chamber view; pulmonary artery velocity waveforms are recorded in the conventional echocardiographic short-axis view. Doppler sample volumes (0.1–0.3 cm) should be placed in the great vessels immediately distal to the semilunar valves. Here, too, the interrogation angle should always be kept at 20° or less. At 11–12 weeks, peak and time-averaged flow velocities are lower than observed in late pregnancy [19], with mean values of 32.1 ± 5.4 cm/s and 11.2 ± 2.2 cm/s in the ascending aorta and 29.6 ± 5.1 cm/s and 10.8 ± 2.1 cm/s in the pulmonary artery [22]. Peak velocities at outflow tract level were also reported by Sharkey et al. [18], who measured a mean peak velocity of 30.2 (± 5.4) cm/s at 13 weeks without differentiating between ascending aorta and pulmonary artery. In both vessels a gestational age-related rise in peak velocities can be demonstrated during the early second trimester of pregnancy, with highest velocities in the ascending aorta [25]. Products of time–velocity integrals and heart rate recorded from all four cardiac valves demonstrate a rise with advancing gestational age, suggesting an increase in cardiac output. A difference in left and right cardiac blood flow in favour of the right side was calculated during the first half of the second trimester of pregnancy. It should be realized, however, that no data are available on foetal blood pressure and venous and arterial volume flow in the late first trimester. It is, therefore, unknown how umbilical–placental resistance precisely affects cardiac flow velocity waveforms at this stage of pregnancy. The higher peak systolic velocities in the ascending aorta compared with the pulmonary artery may be a result of a difference in semilunar valve area between the two vessels, as has been suggested on the basis of similar findings in late pregnancy [1]. Alternatively, a relatively low foetal cerebral vascular resistance with subsequently a lower afterload to the left ventricle may be responsible for the aforementioned difference. The latter seems more likely, since a marked drop in PI has been established in both the foetal descending aorta and umbilical artery at 12–14 weeks of gestation [21, 23] compared with the constantly present low PI values at cerebral level [23].

Extra-cardiac Venous Velocity Waveforms

Flow velocity waveforms from the inferior vena cava can be obtained in a saggital view which includes the foetal right atrium, right ventricle and ascending aorta. The sample volume is positioned over the inferior vena cava immediately proximal to the right atrium [24]. As in late pregnancy, the waveform is characterized by a systolic and early diastolic forward component and a late diastolic retrograde component [7, 16]. Percentage reverse flow at 11-12 weeks is as high as 25%–30%, which is approximately sixfold of that seen in late third trimester pregnancies [7, 16]. A low cardiac compliance or decreased ventricular relaxation rate may be responsible for these high retrograde flow velocities. An association of increased reverse flow with pulsations in the umbilical vein was reported by Rizzo et al. [17], suggesting a relationship between these waveform characteristics and cardiac filling patterns. Umbilical vein pulsations observed in first trimester pregnancies may reflect a high placental resistance, also demonstrated by the high PI values at umbilical artery level at this stage of pregnancy [21, 23].

The ductus venosus, which macroscopically resembles a continuation of the intra-abdominal part of the umbilical vein, joins the inferior vena cava close to the right atrium. The vessel can often not be visualized in late first trimester pregnancies [9]. However, by placing the sample volume immediately above the umbilical sinus, visualized on a transverse cross-sectional view, waveforms can be accepted as originating from this vessel on the basis of their similarity to ductus

cm/s

10 −

0 −

10 −

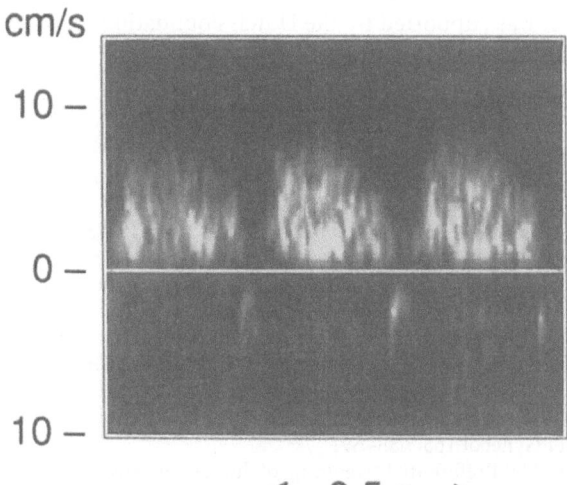

◀   0.5 s   ▶

Fig. 5. Foetal ductus venosus flow velocity waveforms at 9 weeks of gestation

venosus waveforms observed in late pregnancy [8, 12]. Waveforms from the ductus venosus are characterized by a systolic and early diastolic forward component without a late diastolic reverse component. Ductus venosus velocity waveforms may be recorded as early as 9–10 weeks of gestation (Fig. 5). A clear systolic and early diastolic component will become visible as from 11–12 weeks, with peak velocities reaching 30 cm/s at 12 weeks [9]. Time-averaged velocity in the ductus venosus is approximately three times higher than that in the inferior vena cava and umbilical vein [9]. Differences in flow velocities in these venous vessels may result in a tendency not to mix and, therefore, support the idea of preferential streaming of ductus venosus blood flow towards the foramen ovale, as was demonstrated in the foetal lamb [5] and in the human foetus during late gestation [13].

Conclusion

Transvaginal Doppler techniques allow detailed information on foetal waveform characteristics and velocities as early as 8–9 weeks of gestation. Colour-coded Doppler simplifies visualization of foetal vessels of interest. Present flow velocity studies suggest the presence of a high foetal placental vascular resistance in normal late first trimester pregnancy, followed by a marked reduction in resistance in early second trimester pregnancy. Complete dislocation of the trophoblastic plugs at this stage of pregnancy may be responsible for the observed haemodynamic changes.

Doppler studies in early pregnancy provide important information on foetal hemodynamics. Its clinical relevance at this early stage of gestation still needs to be determined.

Acknowledgement. This work was supported by the Dutch Foundation for Medical Research MEDIGON (grant no. 900-568-215).

References

1. Allan LD, Chita SK, Al-Ghazali W, Crowford DC, Tynan M (1987) Doppler echocardiographic evaluation of the normal human fetal heart. Br Heart J 57: 528–533
2. Arduini D, Rizzo G (1991) Umbilical artery velocity waveforms in early pregnancy: a transvaginal color Doppler study. J Clin Ultrasound 19: 335–339
3. Den Ouden M, Cohen-Overbeek TE, Wladimiroff JW (1990) Uterine and fetal umbilical artery flow velocity waveforms in normal first trimester pregnancies. Br J Obstet Gynaecol 97: 716–719
4. Dolkart LA, Reimers FT (1991) Transvaginal fetal echocardiography in early pregnancy: normative data. Am J Obstet Gynecol 165: 688–691
5. Edelstone DI, Rudolph AM (1979) Preferential streaming of ductus venosus blood to the brain and heart in fetal lambs. Am J Physiol 327: H724–H729
6. Guzman ER, Schulman H, Karmel B, Higgins P (1990) Umbilical artery Doppler velocimetry in pregnancies of less than 21 weeks' duration. J Ultrasound Med 9: 655–659
7. Huisman TWA, Stewart PA, Wladimiroff JW (1991) Flow velocity waveforms in the fetal inferior vena cava during the second half of normal pregnancy. Ultrasound Med Biol 17: 679–682
8. Huisman TWA, Stewart PA, Wladimiroff JW (1992) Ductus venosus blood flow velocity waveforms in the human fetus; a Doppler study. Ultrasound Med Biol 18: 33–37
9. Huisman TWA, Stewart PA, Wladimiroff JW (1993) Flow velocity waveforms in the ductus venosus, umbilical vein and inferior vena cava in normal fetuses at 12–15 weeks' gestation. Ultrasound Med Biol 19: 441–445
10. Jauniaux E, Jurkovic D, Campbell S (1991) In vivo investigations of the anatomy and the physiology of early human placental circulations. Ultrasound Obstet Gynecol 1: 435–445
11. Jauniaux E, Jurkovic D, Campbell S, Hustin J (1992) Doppler ultrasound features of the developing placental circulation: correlation with anatomic findings. Am J Obstet Gynecol 166: 585–587
12. Kiserud T, Eik-Nes SH, Blaas HGK, Hellevik LR (1991) Ultrasonographic velocimetry of the fetal ductus venosus. Lancet 338: 1412–1414
13. Kiserud T, Eik-Nes SH, Blaas HGK, Hellevik LR (1992) Foramen ovale, an ultrasonographic study of its relationship to the inferior vena cava, ductus venosus and hepatic veins. Ultrasound Obstet Gynecol 2: 389–397
14. Kurjak A, Jurkovic D, Alfirevic Z, Zalud I (1990) Transvaginal color Doppler imaging. J Clin Ultrasound 18: 227–234
15. Pijnenburg R, Dixon G, Robertson WB, Brosens I (1980) Trophoblastic invasion of human decidua from 8 to 18 weeks of pregnancy. Placenta 1: 3–19
16. Reed KL, Appleton CP, Anderson CF, Shenker L, Sahn DJ (1990) Doppler studies of vena cava flows in human fetuses. Insight into normal and abnormal cardiac physiology. Circulation 81: 498–505
17. Rizzo G, La Marca N, Caforio L, Arduini D (1991) Venous blood flow in early gestation. 5th international fetal cardiology symposium, Rome, 26 Nov., abstract book, p 56
18. Sharkey A, Tulzer G, Huhta J (1991) Doppler blood velocities in the first trimester of pregnancy. Am J Obstet Gynecol 164: 331 (abstract 312)
19. Van der Mooren K, Barendregt LG, Wladimiroff JW (1991) Fetal atrioventricular and outflow tract flow velocity waveforms during the normal second half of pregnancy. Am J Obstet Gynecol 165: 668–674

20. Wladimiroff JW, Seelen JC (1972) Doppler tachometry in early pregnancy. Development of fetal vagal function. Eur J Obstet Gynaecol Reprod Biol 2: 55–63
21. Wladimiroff JW, Huisman TWA, Stewart PA (1991) Fetal and umbilical flow velocity waveforms between 10 and 16 weeks of gestation; a preliminary study. Obstet Gynecol 78: 812–814
22. Wladimiroff JW, Huisman TWA, Stewart PA (1991) Cardiac Doppler flow velocities in the late first trimester feus; a transvaginal Doppler study. J Am Coll Cardiol 17: 1357–1359
23. Wladimiroff JW, Huisman TWA, Stewart PA (1992) Intracerebral, aortic and umbilical artery flow velocity waveforms in the late first trimester fetus. Am J Obstet Gynecol 166: 46–49
24. Wladimiroff JW, Huisman TWA, Stewart PA, Stijnen T (1992) Normal fetal Doppler inferior vena cava, transtricuspid and umbilical artery flow velocity waveforms between 11 and 16 weeks' gestation. Am J Obstet Gynecol 166: 921–924
25. Wladimiroff JW, Stewart PA, Burghouwt MT, Stijnen T (1992) Normal fetal cardiac flow velocity waveforms between 11 and 16 weeks of gestation. Am J Obstet Gynecol 167: 736–739

Transvaginal Examination of the Foetal Heart

G. SHARLAND

Introduction

Congenital heart disease is one of the most common forms of congenital malformation affecting approximately 8 per 1000 live births. Foetal echocardiography has become well established as a means of examining cardiac structures in utero, and as a result most forms of structural cardiac lesion have now been detected during foetal life [2]. However, the antenatal diagnosis of congenital heart disease is rarely made before 16 weeks of gestation using a transabdominal approach. The development of transvaginal ultrasonography has enabled more detailed imaging of foetal anatomy possible in the first trimester of pregnancy [6]. Thus, using high-frequency transducers, it has become possible to detect foetal malformations earlier in pregnancy [4, 12, 13, 17].

Many centres are now using a high-frequency transvaginal transducer to examine the foetal heart [5, 10]. Some studies have shown that the best visualisation of cardiac structures during the early weeks of pregnancy is obtained transvaginally [7]. By this method the highest resolution is between the 11th and 14th week of pregnancy. Between the 15th and 18th week, transvaginal and transabdominal sonography both offer equal advantages. However, after the 19th week of gestation the transabdominal approach appears to be better.

Examination of the Normal Foetal Heart

The cardiac structures to identify are the same whether a transvaginal or transabdominal probe is used. Although the approach to the foetus may be different, the sections sought to examine the foetal heart are still the same. The connections of the heart are most easily seen by obtaining a four-chamber view and then seeking the origin of the two great arteries. The pulmonary and systemic venous connections can also be identified.

Four-Chamber View

The four-chamber view is achieved in a horizontal section of the foetal thorax just above the diaphragm. An example from a foetus at 13 weeks of gestation is shown

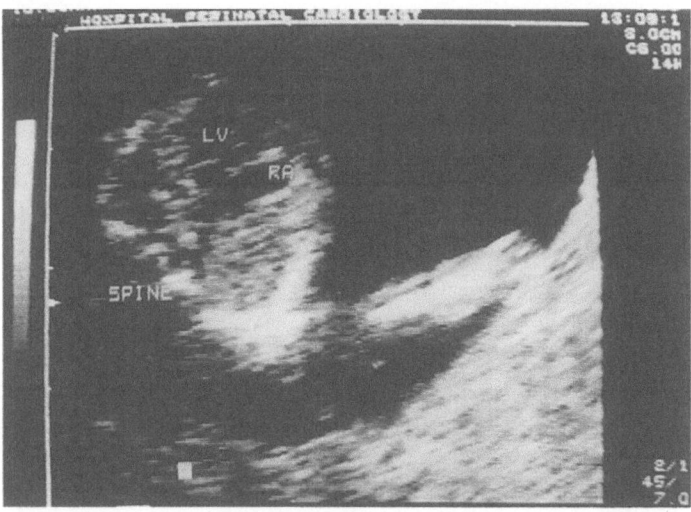

Fig. 1. The four-chamber view of the foetal heart seen at 13 weeks' gestation using a transvaginal transducer. One of the pulmonary veins can be see to be draining into the back of the left atrium. *LV*, left ventricle; *RA*, right atrium

in Fig. 1. The appearance of the four-chamber view will vary according to he orientation of the foetus to the ultrasound beam, but the important points to note are as follows:

1. The heart occupies about a third of the thorax.
2. There are two atria of approximately equal size.
3. There are two ventricles of approximately equal size and thickness. Both show equal contraction in the moving image.
4. The atrial and ventricular septa meet the two atrio-ventricular valves at the crux of the heart in an offset cross.
5. Two opening atrio-ventriclar valves are seen in the moving image.

In addition, scanning up and down horizontally at the back of the left atrium will demonstrate the pulmonary venous connections, as can be seen in Fig. 1.

Imaging the Great Arteries

The two great arteries can be imaged in a variety of projections. Angulating the transducer cranially from the four-chamber view, the aorta can be identified arising from the left ventricle. Figure 2 shows an example of this from a 13-week-old foetus using a transvaginal approach. Transducer angulation in the other direction will allow the right heart connections to be seen. Alternatively, making a horizontal section across the foetal thorax, more cranially than the four-chamber view allows identification of the pulmonary artery and arterial duct. This is illustrated in a 13-week-old foetus, using the transvaginal approach, in Fig. 3. The aortic arch can also

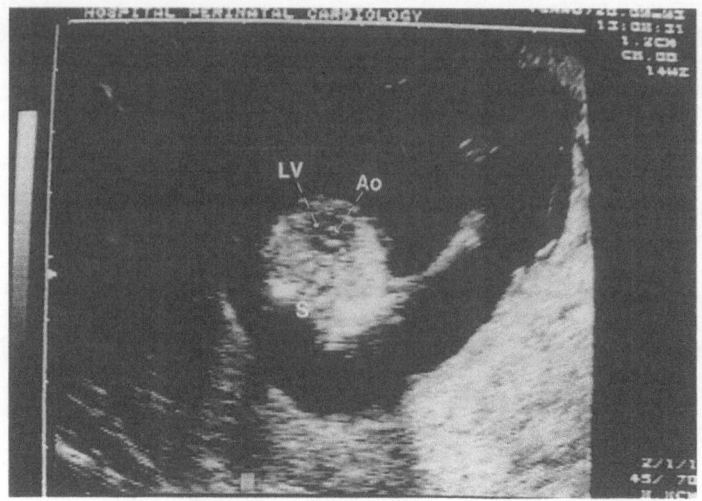

Fig. 2. The aorta in a 13-week-old foetus can be seen to be arising from the left ventricle (*LV*) and is directed towards the right shoulder. *Ao*, aorta; *S*, spine

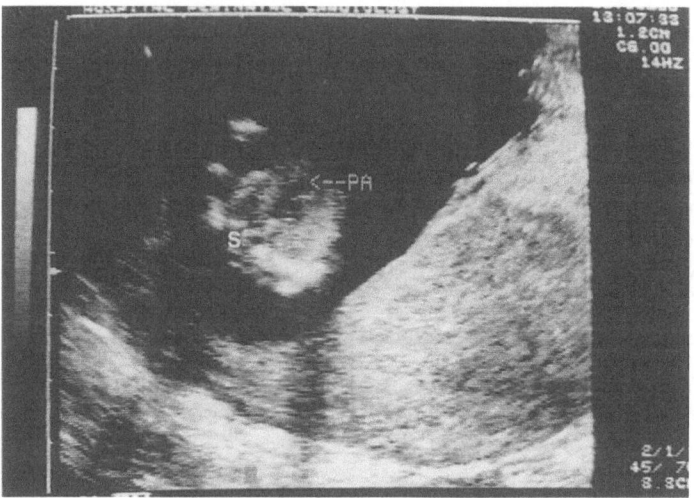

Fig. 3. The pulmonary artery (*PA*) in a 13-week-old foetus can be seen arising anteriorly and directed towards the spine (*S*)

be imaged in a longitudinal section of the foetus. The aorta normally arises in the centre of the thorax and forms a tight hook shape, with the head and neck vessels arising from the crest of the arch (Figure 4).

The important features to note when examining the great arteries are as follows:

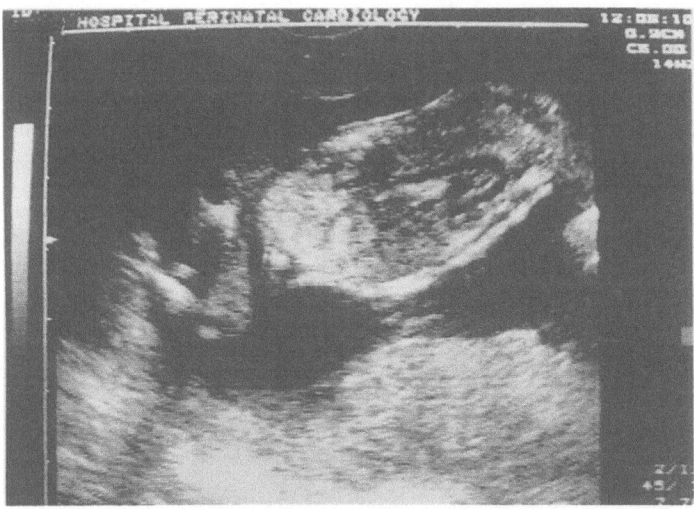

Fig. 4. The aortic arch and descending aorta in a 13-week-old foetus are seen in a longitudinal projection

1. Two arterial valves can always be seen.
2. The aorta arises wholly from the left ventricle.
3. The great arteries are similar in size, but the pulmonary artery at the valve ring is slightly bigger than the aorta.
4. The pulmonary valve is anterior and cranial to the aortic valve.
5. At their origins the great arteries lie at right angles to, and cross over, each other.
6. The arch of the aorta is of similar size to the pulmonary artery and duct and is complete.

Use of Colour Doppler

The majority of structural cardiac defects can be diagnosed by the real-time cross-sectional image. The addition of Doppler and colour Doppler to the study can help in the precision of diagnosis [1, 15]. The usefulness of transvaginal flow imaging in the assessment of foetal heart and haemodynamics has also been reported [16].

Colour flow imaging allows normal and abnormal patterns of blood flow to be identified in the fetal cardiovascular system. The direction of flow is best seen when the line of flow is parallel to the ultrasonic beam, although some flow can be identified at other angles. The cardiac flow patterns detected with a transvaginal probe are the same as those detected with a transabdominal probe. It should be possible to identify the inflow across the two atrio-ventricular valves and the outflow across the two arterial valves and through the arterial duct. Flow across the two atrio-ventricular valves can be compared in a four-chamber view and should

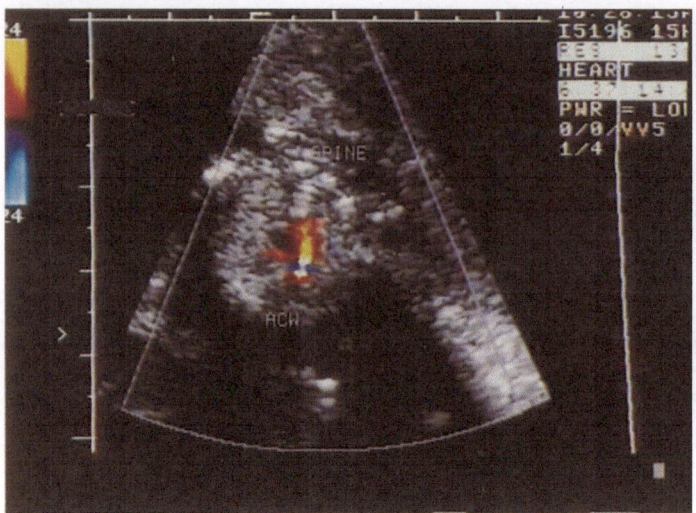

Fig. 5. Colour Doppler identifies the pulmonary artery arising beneath the anterior chest wall (*ACW*) in a foetus of 14 weeks' gestation. This vessel is directed towards the spine as it joins the ductal connection and descending aorta

appear equal on both sides. The colour flow map can identify the two great arteries at their origin and can also demonstrate their relative size and course in the upper thorax, in the aortic arch and in the arterial duct.

The ease with which cardiac structures can be identified with colour flow imaging improves with experience. When scanning the foetal heart in the first trimester, it can be difficult to correctly identify all the cardiac structures. This is particularly true of the great arteries, which may only measure 1–2 mm. The use of colour flow imaging can help to identify these with more confidence. An example of this is illustrated in Fig. 5, where the pulmonary artery and duct in a 14-week-old foetus are clearly shown with colour flow imaging. Indeed, Gembruch et al. [10] found that, in a series of 114 fetuses scanned between 11–16 weeks of pregnancy, they were able to identify the four-chamber view and the origin of the two great arteries in all cases from the 13th week of pregnancy. The high success rate in this study appears to be related to the use of colour Doppler to identify the great arteries. In contrast, Dolkart and Reimers [8] reported 52 transvaginal scans performed between 10 and 14.9 weeks of pregnancy. They were able to identify the four-chamber view in 90% of foetuses at 12 weeks of gestation and in 100% by 13 weeks of gestation. In the study reported by Dolkart and Reimers, the arterial connections could only be identified in 30%. Johnson et al. [11] were able to identify the four-chamber view in only 74% of foetuses at 13 weeks of gestation. However, no colour flow imaging was used in this study, and the time allowed for each scan, which also included examination of other foetal anatomy, was 10 min. These are probably the main reasons why the success rate in this particular study was less than in others.

Detection of Cardiac Abnormalities

When the operator is familiar with normal patterns of flow within the cardiovascular system, colour Doppler can be helpful in the accurate definition of cardiac anomalies in the foetus. Absence of flow across atretic valves, turbulent flow across stenosed valves and regurgitant through abnormal valves can easily be detected with colour flow studies. The use of colour flow imaging usually confirms abnormalities already suspected on cross-sectional imaging, but may occasionally lead to the detection of an abnormality not previously obvious.

One of the earliest reported diagnoses of congenital heart disease in the foetus was by Gembruch et al. in 1990 [9]. The diagnosis of a complete atrio-ventricular septal defect with atrio-ventricular valve insufficiency, in association with complete heart block, was made in a foetus of 11 weeks' gestation using transvaginal echocardiography. The foetus also had non-immune hydrops fetalis. In the same year, Bronshtein et al. [3] reported the early diagnosis of an isolated ventricular septal defect and of a ventricular septal defect associated with an overriding aorta, again using transvaginal echocardiography.

In 1993, Gembruch et al. [10] reported a series of 13 foetal cardiac malformations detected by transvaginal echocardiography between the 11th and 16th weeks of gestation. In the majority of cases the major cardiac lesion was correctly made, but in one case the diagnosis of an atrio-ventricular septal defect was incorrectly made, and in a further case the diagnosis of an atrio-ventricular septal defect with a double outlet right ventricle was not made until 21 weeks of gestation. In all except one case, the indication for foetal echocardiography was the detection of an extra-cardiac fetal anomaly. The remaining case had a family history of congenital heart disease.

In a much larger series of 12 793 transvaginal ultrasound examinations between 12–16 weeks of gestation, Bronshtein et al. (1993) detected 47 foetuses with congenital heart disease. In this series 27% of women scanned were high risk for foetal congenital heart defects. The remaining 73% were a low-risk population. Of the cardiac abnormalities detected, 29 occurred in the low-risk group. However, 62% of the foetuses with cardiac anomalies had an extra-cardiac anomaly and 36% had a karyotypic abnormality.

Thus, it is now quite clear that the diagnosis of foetal congenital heart disease can be made in the first trimester of pregnancy. Many centres have found that the addition of transvaginal colour flow imaging adds to the accuracy of diagnosis. However, the majority of cardiac abnormalities detected in the first trimester have been detected in foetuses with additional extra-cardiac anomalies. In most centres, the detection rate for isolated cardiac lesions is still low compared with transabdominal echocardiography. This is most likely related to the fact that most cases of foetal congenital heart disease will occur in a low-risk population. The detection of these cases has increased as a result of screening during routine obstetric scans [14]. Unless transvaginal scanning becomes a part of routine obstetric scanning, the antenatal diagnosis of the majority of cases of congenital heart disease will still be made in the second and third trimesters of pregnancy. Even so, there is still a definite role for transvaginal echocardiography in high-risk groups, as there are many benefits of first-trimester diagnosis of cardiac malformations. There is the additional benefit of being able to provide earlier reassurance to parents who have lost a previous child with heart disease.

Limitations

Although there are many advantages provided by the use of transvaginal transducers, the disadvantages also need consideration. Most pregnant women will find this method of examination acceptable, but some women may refuse it.

There is a greater restriction in scanning in all planes compared to transabdominal transducers. This is due to the narrow focal range and the limited mobility of the transducer. An unfavourable foetal position will make it much more difficult to visualise the foetal heart compared with transabdominal scanning. The small size of the foetal heart will make the detection of some forms of heart disease much more difficult in the first trimester of pregnancy.

The most important aspect that must always be remembered is that of safety. The effects of ultrasound and the hazards of Doppler, particularly in the first trimester of pregnancy, are still unknown. It would therefore be prudent to restrict the use of Doppler to high-risk cases and in particular to those cases where it is likely to provide additional useful information.

References

1. Allan LD, Chita SK, Al-Ghazali W, Crawford DC, Tynan MJ (1987) Doppler echocardiographic evaluation of the normal human fetal heart. Br Heart J 57: 528–533
2. Allan LD, Chita SK, Sharland GK, Fagg N, Anderson RH, Crawford DC (1989) The accuracy of fetal echocardiography in the diagnosis of CHD. Int J Cardiol 25: 279–288
3. Bronshtein M, Sieglar E, Yoffe N, Zimmer EZ (1990) The prenatal diagnosis of ventricular septal defect and overriding aorta at 14 weeks' gestation using transvaginal sonography. Prenat Diagn 10: 697–702
4. Bronshtein M, Zimmer EZ, Milo S, Ho SY, Lorber A, Gerlis LM (1991) Fetal cardiac abnormalities detected by transvaginal sonography at 12–16 weeks' gestation. Am J Obstet Gynecol 78: 374–378
5. Bronshtein M, Zimmer EZ, Gerlis LM, Lorber A, Drugan A (1993) Early ultrasound diagnosis of fetal congenital heart defects in high-risk and low-risk pregnancies. Obstet Gynecol 82: 225–229
6. Cullen NT, Green J, Whethen J, Salafia C, Gabriella S, Haggins JC (1990) Transvaginal ultrasonographic detection of congenital anomalies in the first trimester. Am J Obstet Gynecol 163: 466–476
7. D'Amelio R, Giorlandino C, Masala L, Garafalo M, Martinelli M, Anelli G, Zichella L (1991) Fetal echocardiography using transvaginal and transabdominal probes during the first period of pregnancy: a comparative study. Prenat Diagn 11: 69–75
8. Dolkart LA, Reimers FT (1991) Transvaginal fetal echocardiography in early pregnancy: normative data. Am J Obstet Gynecol 165: 688–691

9. Gembruch U, Knopfle G, Chatterjee M, Bald R, Hansmann M (1990) First trimester diagnosis of fetal congenital heart disease by transvaginal two-dimensional and Doppler echocardiography. Obstet Gynecol 75: 496–498

10. Gembruch U, Knopfle G, Bold R, Hansmann M (1993) Early diagnosis of fetal congenital heart disease by transvaginal echocardiography. Ultrasound Obstet Gynecol 3: 310–317

11. Johnson P, Sharland G, Maxwell D, Allan L (1992) The role of transvaginal sonography in the early detection of congenital heart disease. Ultrasound Obstet Gynecol 2: 248–251

12. Quashie C, Weiner S, Bolognese R (1992) Efficacy of first trimester transvaginal sonography in detecting normal fetal development. Am J Perinat 9: 209–213

13. Rottem S, Bronshtein M (1990) Transvaginal sonographic diagnosis of congenital anomalies between 9 weeks and 16 weeks menstrual age. J Clin Ultrasound 18: 307–314

14. Sharland GK, Allan LD (1992) Screening for congenital heart disease prenatally. Results of a 2½ year study in the South East Thames Region. Br J Obstet Gynaecol 99: 220–225

15. Sharland GK, Chita SK, Allan LD (1990) The use of colour Doppler in fetal echocardiography. Int J Cardiol 28: 229–236

16. Sohda S, Hamada H, Okane M, Mesaki N, Kubo T (1992) Fetal hemodynamics assessed by transvaginal color flow mapping during the first and early second trimesters. Acta Obstet Gynaecol Jpn 44: 1537–1542

17. Timor-Trish IE, Monteagudo A, Peisner DB (1992) High-frequency transvaginal sonographic examination for the potential malformation assessment of the 9 week to 14 week fetus. J Clin Ultrasound 20: 231–238

V. Urinary Tract

Doppler Studies of the Lower Urinary Tract

V. Khullar and L.D. Cardozo

Introduction

Ultrasound of the lower urinary tract poses problems for the sonographer. Clear views of the pelvis through the abdomen rely on the urine-filled bladder to act as an acoustic window and this is useful for delineating bladder tumours [2] and measuring post-void residuals [14]; however, by filling the bladder its structure is difficult to visualise. The retropubic position of the bladder neck and urethra make transvaginal [15], transrectal [17, 18] and transperineal ultrasound [11] the ideal methods of visualising the bladder and urethra. The transabdominal approach does not reliably image the bladder neck and urethra, particularly in the obese or in women suffering genuine stress incontinence. The transvaginal approach, when used to image urinary leakage into the proximal urethra, should be interpreted with caution, as compression of the urethra can occur [19]. The transrectal approach does not alter any urodynamic parameter, but there can be problems in visualising the bladder neck and urethra if a rectocele is present [18]. The transperineal approach has the advantage of direct contact with the distal end of the urethra, and the proximity of the probe ensures good images of the periurethral structures despite vaginal prolapse [9].

Bladder Wall Imaging

The bladder is best imaged transvaginally, not only because the higher ultrasound frequencies needed to image small structures have reduced tissue penetration, but urinary bladder volumes in excess of 50 ml reduce the bladder wall thickness [5]. This makes a transabdominal approach unrewarding. Blood flow measurements within the bladder wall are reduced at volumes greater than 30 ml, thus making it extremely important to ensure that the bladder is emptied. Most women (90%) empty their bladders to less than 10 ml [4], so that catheterisation is not usually necessary. The measurement of bladder wall thickness is performed with the woman supine. The vaginal probe is held at the introitus, and the urethra and bladder are visualised in the midline (Fig. 1). The symphysis pubis has a hyperechoic inferior edge and casts a hypoechoic shadow [16]. The urethra is identified as a hypoechoic area inferior to the symphysis pubis. Bladder wall thickness is measured in a parasagittal plane; as the urethral hypoechoic area

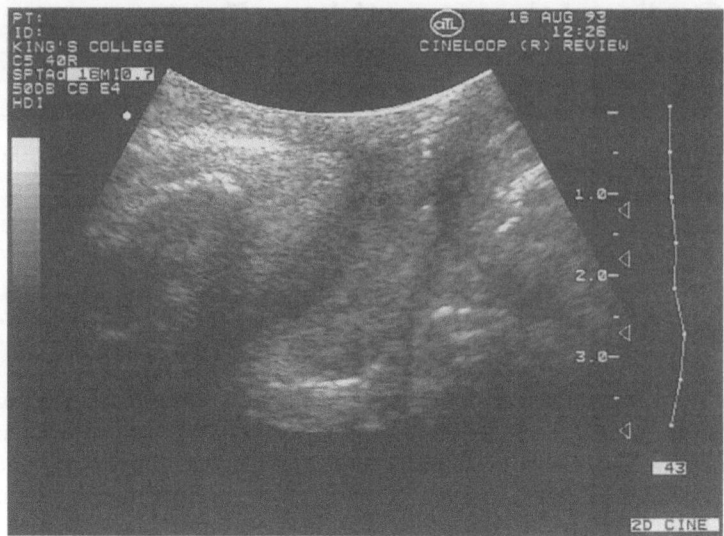

Fig. 1. Transvaginal view of the bladder, urethra and symphysis pubis

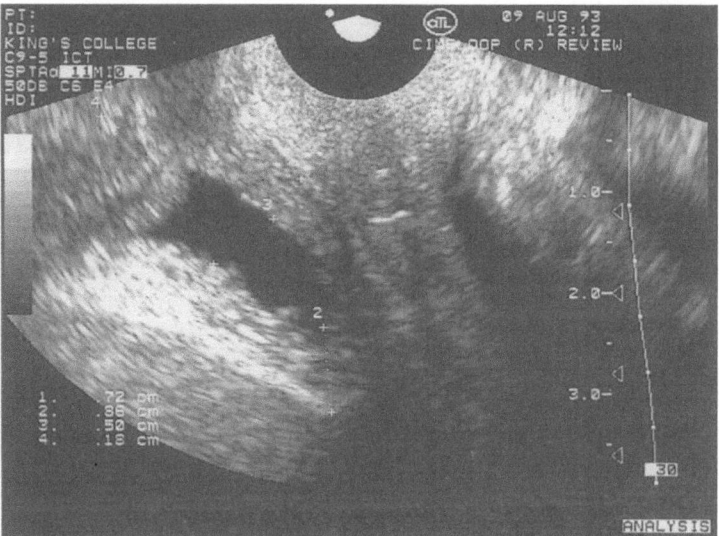

Fig. 2. Parasagittal transvaginal view through the bladder while taking bladder wall thickness measurements

produces a shadow over the dome of the bladder, measurements are taken from the dome of the bladder, anterior bladder wall and trigone (Fig. 2). Care must be taken to measure the thickest part of the bladder wall imaged and measurements must be made perpendicular to the epithelial surface of the bladder.

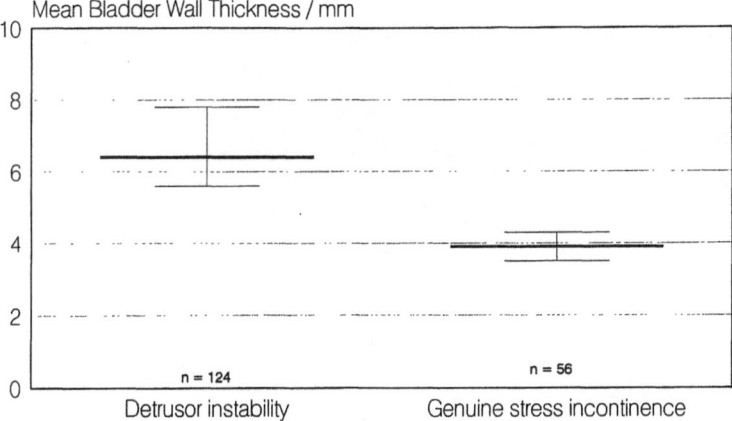

Fig. 3. Mean bladder wall thickness in 180 women compared with urodynamic diagnosis with both videocystourethrography and ambulatory urodynamics

In a study of 180 symptomatic women (Fig. 3), increased bladder wall thickness greater than 5 mm was associated with the presence of detrusor instability diagnosed on videocystourethrography and ambulatory urodynamics in 94% of these women. This may potentially be a sensitive method of detecting detrusor instability, as the activity required to produce detrusor hypertrophy occurs over a long period of time, rather than the urodynamic test, which has a much shorter duration. Severe urethral sphincter incompetence with detrusor instability may not produce detrusor hypertrophy due to the reduced outflow resistance; this poses a diagnostic challenge which will probably require the use of conventional cystometry.

Colour Doppler ureteric jets (Fig. 4) have been studied, and the distance of the ureteric jet origin from the midline has been correlated with reflux; the velocity and longitudinal angle have not been found to be useful [12]. The velocity and frequency of the ureteric jets correlate with the state of hydration of the subject, both increasing with increased hydration.

The trigone, bladder neck and terminal part of the ureter are supplied by the inferior vesical artery. The fundus of the bladder is supplied by the superior vesical artery. Intramural bladder blood flow is measured at the edge of the trigone where the ureters insert. This is easily identified by imaging the ureteric jets of urine entering the bladder on colour Doppler ultrasound. Blood flow has been studied in women suffering urinary incontinence. There are two main urodynamic diagnoses: genuine stress incontinence, where there is an involuntary loss of urine when the intravesical pressure exceeds the maximum urethral closure pressure in the absence of detrusor instability, and detrusor instability, where the detrusor is objectively shown to contract, either spontaneously or on provocation, during bladder filling, while the subject is attempting to inhibit micturition [1].

Colour Doppler ultrasound can detect blood flow in the fundus of the bladder in women with detrusor instability and in young women. In women with genuine

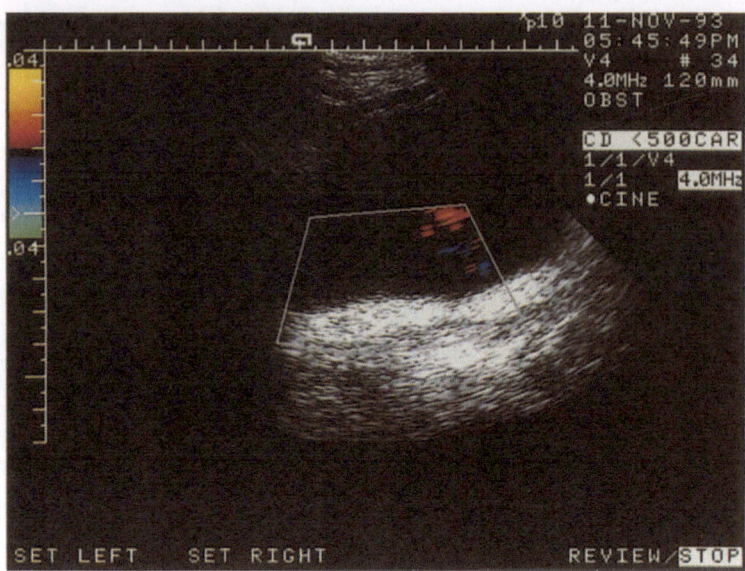

Fig. 4. Sagittal colour Doppler abdominal scan of a full bladder. Urine jetting from ureteral jet into the bladder

stress incontinence, blood flow is rarely seen in the fundus. Intramural blood flow in normal asymptomatic women, women with diagnosed genuine stress incontinence (pulsatility index, PI, 3.21; SD 1.4; $n = 31$) and detrusor instability (PI, 1.74; SD 1.24; $n = 40$) all show little change with age [7, 8].

Women who have been diagnosed as having sensory urgency on cystometry have painful catheterisation and reduced maximum bladder capacities (less than 400 ml) in the absence of detrusor instability. These patients should undergo cystoscopy and bladder wall biopsy. Using transvaginal ultrasound, the bladder wall can be visualised; the detrusor muscle layer appears as a hyperechoic area and the lamina propria as a hypoechoic area [10]. This may be useful in the future for diagnosing inflammatory pathological processes within the bladder wall causing oedema and swelling of the tissues. Colour flow Doppler has been used to image intramural bladder blood flow in these women. If the PI is less than 2.00, then an inflammatory process within the bladder wall should be suspected and cystoscopy and bladder wall biopsy would be useful (Fig. 5). There is no difference on colour flow Doppler between women with chronic follicular cystitis and those with interstitial cystitis: both have increased blood flow.

Imaging of the Urethra and Periurethral Structures

Ultrasound imaging of the urethra and bladder neck is best performed using the transperineal approach rather than the transvaginal route, not only because of

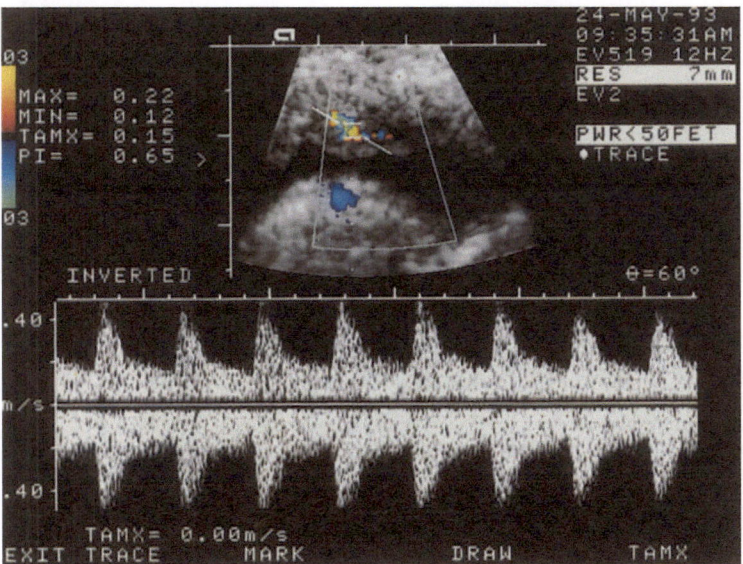

Fig. 5. Transvaginal scan of the bladder wall of a woman with diagnosed sensory urgency on urodynamics; bladder wall biopsy showed chronic follicular cystitis

pressure applied to the urethra by the vaginal probe [19], but also because the probe moves on Valsalva's manoeuvre, making measurements of bladder neck movement difficult, particularly in women with a cystocele.

Colour Doppler blood flow measurement of the inferior vesical artery is performed using the transperineal approach with a 5-MHz ultrasound probe (3.5-MHz ultrasound probes are not adequate). Visualising the urethra and bladder neck in the midline, the probe is directed laterally 15° and the ultrasound probe is rotated until the base of the bladder is seen. The vessel running along the bladder base from the pelvic side walls towards the bladder neck is the inferior vesical artery (Fig. 6). This is a branch of the anterior division of the internal iliac artery, and the velocity waveform has a characteristic notch [6] (Fig. 7). The vessels supplying the urethra and rhabdosphincter appear to be branches of the inferior vesical artery. In young women a large periurethral vascular plexus can be seen which is fed by lateral vessels [13]. Women with genuine stress incontinence have lower peak (13.8 cm/s) and mean velocities (5.8 cm/s) and PI of 1.43 (SD, 0.42) than women with detrusor instability (peak velocity, 16.7 cm/s; mean velocity, 7.1 cm/s; PI, 2.19; SD, 0.99). The reduced blood flow to the bladder neck in women with genuine stress incontinence is reduced further by increasing age and there is a negative correlation with age [7]. This has important implications for medical treatment of genuine stress incontinence. Oestrogen replacement therapy is used to treat genuine stress incontinence. By increasing blood flow to the urethra, oestrogen appears to potentiate the alpha adrenergic receptor agonists. The reduction in blood flow in the inferior vesical artery seen on colour Doppler in some

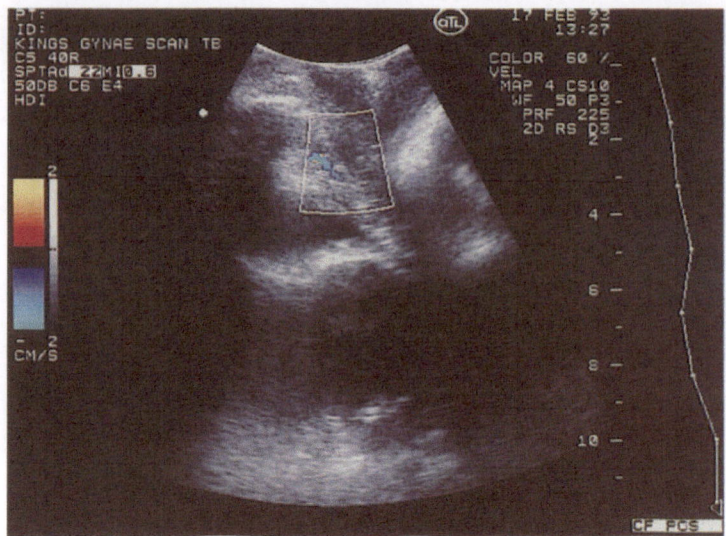

Fig. 6. Perineal scan of the inferior vesical artery

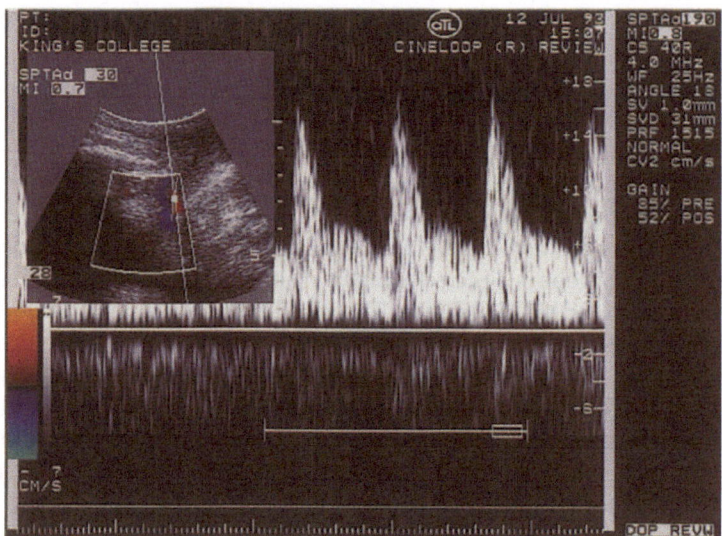

Fig. 7. Velocity waveform of the inferior vesical artery

women with genuine stress incontinence could lead to a reduced response to oestrogen therapy.

It is not surprising that the majority of randomised controlled trials of oestrogen in the treatment of urinary incontinence have not shown significant improvements [3]. Colour Doppler may potentially be useful to determine which

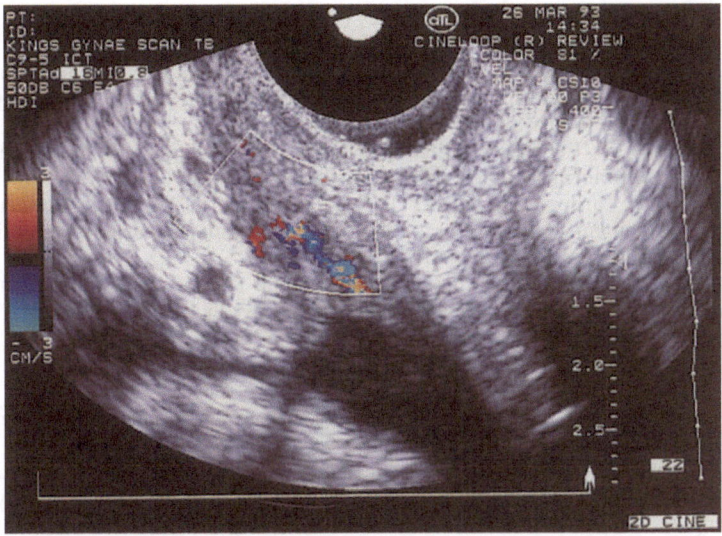

Fig. 8. Increased colour Doppler around urethra in woman with urethritis

women would benefit from oestrogen therapy. Absent or severely damaged urethral blood vessels may not be able to respond to hormone therapy in the same way as normal vasculature. Continent women taking systemic oestrogens have PI less than 1.00, whereas those women with genuine stress incontinence taking systemic oestrogen replacement therapy have PI from 3.78 to 0.80 ($n = 25$). Women with severe urethritis have increased blood flow (Fig. 8) and the PI of the inferior vesical artery is less than one.

In conclusion, this is an exciting new field for which the transvaginal/transperineal approach is ideal. The study of bladder and periurethral blood flow has implications for the assessment of urethral function and may also have benefits in evaluating the efficacy of treatment.

References

1. Abrams P, Blaivas JG, Stanton SL, Andersen JT (1990) The standardisation of terminology of lower urinary tract function. Br J Obstet Gynaecol 6 [Suppl]: 1–16
2. Davies AH, Mastorakou I, Dickinson AJ, Cranston D, O'Kelly TJ, Turner WH, Fellows GJ (1991) Flexible cystoscopy compared with ultrasound in the detection of recurrent bladder tumours. Br J Urol 67: 491–492
3. Fantl JA, Cardozo LD, McClish DK, et al (1994) Estrogen therapy in the management of urinary incontinence in postmenopausal women: a meta-analysis. First report of the Hormones and Urogenital Therapy Committee. Obstet Gynaecol 83: 12–18
4. Haylen BT (1989) Residual urine volumes in a normal female population: application of transvaginal ultrasound. Br J Urol 64: 347–349
5. Khullar V, Cardozo LD, Abbott D, Kelleher CJ (1993a) Changes in bladder wall thickness with fluid volume. Int Urogynaecol J 4: 329

6. Khullar V, Cardozo LD, Bourne TH, Kelleher CJ (1993b) Description and validation of the inferior vesical artery. Ultra Obstet Gynecol 3 [Suppl 1]: 35

7. Khullar V, Cardozo LD, Kelleher CJ, Abbott D, Bourne TH (1993c) Blood flow in the lower urinary tract in women with genuine stress incontinence and detrusor instability. Ultra Obstet Gynecol 3 [Suppl 2]: 105

8. Khullar V, Cardozo LD, Kelleher CJ, Abbott D, Bourne TH (1993d) Blood flow in the lower urinary tract in normal women. Ultra Obstet Gynecol 3 [Suppl 2]: 106

9. Khullar V, Abbott D, Cardozo LD, Kelleher CJ, Salvatore S, Bourne TH (1994a) Perineal ultrasound measurement of the urethral sphincter in women with urinary incontinence: an aid to diagnosis? Br J Radiol 67: 713–714

10. Khullar V, Kelleher CJ, Salvatore S, Boyle M, Cardozo LD (1994b) Ultrasound of the bladder – a replacement for cystoscopy and bladder biopsy? Br J Obstet Gynaecol (in press)

11. Koelbl H, Bernaschek G (1989) A new method for sonographic urethrocystography and simultaneous pressure-flow measurements. Obstet Gynaecol 74: 417–422

12. Marshall JL, Johnson ND, De Campo MP (1990) Vesicoureteric reflux in children: prediction with colour Doppler imaging. Radiology 175: 355–358

13. Mattox TF, Sinow R, Renslo R, Bhatia NN (1992) The physiology of periurethral vasculature using colour flow doppler. Proceedings of the International Continence Society, 22nd Meeting. Halifax 161

14. Poston J, Joseph AEA, Riddle PR (1983) The accuracy of ultrasound in the measurement of changes in bladder volume. Br J Urol 55: 361–363

15. Quinn MJ, Beynon J, Mc Mortensen C, Smith PJB (1988) Transvaginal endosonography: a new method to study the anatomy of the lower urinary tract in urinary stress incontinence. Br J Urol 62: 414–418

16. Quinn MJ (1990) Vaginal ultrasound and urinary stress incontinence. Contemp Rev Obstet Gynaecol 2: 104–110

17. Richmond DH, Sutherst JR, Brown MC (1986) Screening of the bladder base and urethra using linear array transrectal ultrasound scanning. J Clin Ultrasound 14: 647–651

18. Richmond DH, Sutherst J (1989) Transrectal ultrasound scanning in urinary incontinence: the effect of the probe on urodynamic parameters. Br J Urol 64: 582–585

19. Wise BG, Burton G, Cutner A, Cardozo LD (1992) Effect of vaginal ultrasound probe on lower urinary tract function. Br J Urol 70: 12–16

Subject Index

Springer-Verlag
and the Environment

We at Springer-Verlag firmly believe that an international science publisher has a special obligation to the environment, and our corporate policies consistently reflect this conviction.

We also expect our business partners – paper mills, printers, packaging manufacturers, etc. – to commit themselves to using environmentally friendly materials and production processes.

The paper in this book is made from low- or no-chlorine pulp and is acid free, in conformance with international standards for paper permanency.